You are passionate
about family
nursing care.
Enjoy,
Veryl

NO NEED *TO*
TROUBLE
THE HEART

NO NEED *TO* TROUBLE *THE* HEART

PATRICK CONLON

Foreword by June Callwood

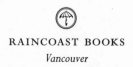

RAINCOAST BOOKS

Vancouver

Raincoast Books gratefully acknowledges the ongoing support of the
Canada Council for the Arts, the British Columbia Arts Council and
the Government of Canada through the Book Publishing Industry
Development Program (BPIDP).

Edited by Steven Beattie
Cover and interior design by Teresa Bubela

Library and Archives Canada Cataloguing in Publication
Conlon, Patrick, 1944-
No need to trouble the heart / Patrick Conlon.

ISBN 10: 1-55192-875-2
ISBN 13: 978-1-55192-875-3

1. Hospital patients—Family relationships. 2. Health care teams.
3. Conlon, Patrick, 1944-. 4. O'Neill, Jim. 5. Hospital patients—Ontario.
6. Hospital care—Ontario. I. Title.
RA965.6.C65 2006   362.11   C2005-905458-1

Raincoast Books
9050 Shaughnessy Street
Vancouver, British Columbia
Canada V6P 6E5
www.raincoast.com

Raincoast Books is committed to protecting the environment and to the
responsible use of natural resources. We are working with suppliers and
printers to phase out our use of paper produced from ancient forests.
This book is printed with vegetable-based inks on 100% ancient-forest-
free paper, processed chlorine- and acid-free. For further information,
visit our website at www.raincoast.com/publishing.

Printed in Canada by Friesens.

10 9 8 7 6 5 4 3 2 1

For Jim, of course

CONTENTS

ACKNOWLEDGEMENTS

Writers can be fond of whining about the solitary nature of their work. Don't be fooled.

While books like this are finally down to a single pair of hands, a keyboard and a deadline, they really emerge from a chorus of voices.

Donna Butt nudged me to start writing this story. I told her she was nuts, and then started. Roger Abbott, Andy Barrie, June Callwood, Michele Landsberg, Rob Sheppard and Penny Williams inspired me to keep going when giving up seemed sensible. Samantha Haywood found a good home for the book, proving in the process she's not only smart and beautiful but a splendid literary agent as well. And editor Steven Beattie helped bring clarity and depth to the final manuscript, pressing gently but relentlessly for a better book, followed by copyeditor Helen Godolphin whose keen eyes missed nothing. I'm deeply grateful to all of them.

Family and friends and neighbours who stepped forward to offer food and support and sympathy and sometimes just their ears were never taken for granted and will never be forgotten.

Many of them moved me to tears with their open hearts. Together, they showed that "community" isn't just a slogan.

Dr. Tom Stewart and senior respiratory therapist Rod MacDonald at Mount Sinai Hospital ICU shared invaluable medical information with great patience and generosity. Advice from Dr. Sue Comay and her colleagues at Vancouver's Pine Clinic was very beneficial in framing the clinical details of Jim's diagnosis. The wonderful Dr. Margaret Herridge of Toronto's University Health Network and Eileen Rubin Zacharias of The ARDS Foundation (www.ardsil.com) both helped illuminate acute respiratory distress syndrome (ARDS), a baffling condition that even with diagnostic and treatment advances remains an equal-opportunity killer. No one is immune.

Through Jim's long hospital stay, I was privileged to work alongside more than a hundred nurses. I have great respect for all the skilled doctors who attended Jim but I quickly learned that nurses are the ones who do the heavy lifting. All were dedicated and compassionate allies in Jim's care, and I thank them — but I have to single out the exceptional nursing and therapy teams in Mount Sinai ICU and Trillium Med 4D. They actively encouraged me to join them as they cared for Jim, and they extended the invitation with grace and wisdom.

It's break time. Coffee and doughnuts are on me.

FOREWORD

by June Callwood

I nto every imagination, a certain terror arises from a deep place and feels so real that tears sting the eyes. It comes in tender moments of a relationship between parent and child, between an adult and an ageing parent, between all people who are well-and-dearly mated. Out of blue sky, the person is struck by love so intense and stabbing that dread of loss comes along with it. "What if this irreplaceable one dies," an inner voice mutters. "Could you stand it?" *No.*

Then, one appalling day, the beloved one is close to death. Nurses and doctors speak in a softened tone of voice, like undertakers do, as they relay numbing details about the condition and the prognosis. What filters through pain is their alarming uncertainty. If this happens, and if that doesn't ... The vigil begins. Hospitals at night are usually accommodating of those in grief who will not leave. Time, which rules the world, doesn't enter the ghastly space around the sick person. Check the clock and it is noon; a few minutes later comes the noise of the cart bearing dinner trays and, surprisingly, it is dusk outside. Where did those hours go? The world is constricted: nothing exists but the motionless person in the high hospital bed, and horror.

Patrick Conlon, a friend and colleague of mine, endured such agony and wrote this moving book about it. The person who was lying in an island of life-supports was his beloved partner of thirty years, Jim O'Neill.

The generation now entering adulthood cannot know what used to be common practice when same-sex couples were hit with a medical crisis. Very often, health professionals and family barred access to the sick one's mate and made no effort to hide their dislike. Decisions about care, which in heterosexual couples are directed as a matter of right to the spouse, were instead made without the same-sex spouse's involvement. Stories abounded of funeral arrangements which left out the partner, and even directives that the partner stay away from the burial.

Canadians are in the process of enlightened growth; in fact, observably and to our eternal credit, we now are world leaders in acceptance of diversity. Just three years ago, however, Patrick could not be sure of his welcome in the Intensive Care Unit when Jim fell gravely ill. If he were excluded, as had happened with many gay couples he knew, he could not imagine how he would handle it.

What happened instead was almost as blessed a miracle as Jim's eventual recovery. The relationship between Patrick and Jim was recognized for what it was: two adults who had a deep commitment to one another. Their sexual orientation was as irrelevant as their eye colour. Jim received compassionate care, and the healing constant presence of a loving, articulate, informed and watchful partner.

Patrick's book is one of such embracing sweetness that it made me weep. The men saw each other through the kind of nightmare we all fear most. Their story is more than an inspiration. It's a gift.

— *June Callwood*

ONE

*E*arly one Monday morning just before Christmas, while the wind roused a chunky vine to rap insistently on the window like a mischievous friend, Jim settled into his favourite chair and began to die.

That was not the plan. We had talked the night before, and the plan was to sleep and then to visit the local walk-in clinic next morning. We would stroll in and wait tolerantly for attention while we thumbed old magazines. It would be our first time there but it seemed like a good idea because a lingering bout of flu had left him short of breath, and he complained he was sore around his rib cage. It was probably just muscle strain from all the coughing, he mumbled, or a residual infection, and I wanted to believe him. We were rational adults. Antibiotics and sleep could fix this. And I could imagine that his occasional hallucinations, his distressed certainty at times that there were other people in the room with us, were only transient side effects that would yield to a doctor's expedient attention, fading into memory as he recovered. There was nothing to fear.

He was feeble and shaky but he had managed to dress himself with slow deliberation in comfortable sweatpants and he had humped down the stairs to the living room on his backside, obstinately rejecting any help, the evidence of independence encouraging. He had a nice view of the benign December sky, with music about triumph and joy playing gently on the stereo and a box of decorations on the coffee table next to the unsent Christmas cards, but I was now becoming certain that the chair was as far as he could go without help, that he had exhausted himself, and the realization frightened me.

But we would not be alone. Donna had offered to accompany us to the clinic and I called her, determined to hold to the plan, to pretend that a cure was a short car ride away. She's a veteran nurse and a friend, she lives down the street, she had not seen him for a week but we had talked every day and she had recommended Gatorade through the worst of his flu to keep his electrolytes up and she knows staff at the clinic. Maybe we could even jump the line. Besides, her four-door car is an easier in and out than ours. But I asked her to have a quick look at him before we all left, to summon those assessment skills that come naturally to experienced nurses. Finally, I could no longer resist the nagging dread that something terribly wrong was unfolding, that a feral and relentless predator had not finished its awful work on him and that he and I were fools to think it had. But just then I wanted complicity in our defiance. I wanted Donna to appraise him and say cheerfully, "Okay, let's go." She was at our door in minutes.

She squinted down at Jim, now perspiring and agitated, still fighting for air. She frowned and shook her head, her eyes on him but speaking quietly to me and failing to mask her obvious shock. "I think he's in bad shape," she said. "I don't think the walk-in clinic is an option. I think we should call 9-1-1. Want me to do it?" Without waiting for response, she left to use the phone in the kitchen.

I started to follow her, then stopped, caught between Jim and her, and I overheard one of those terse conversations that mellow urgency with an overlay of professional calm. "No," Donna said, "he's not cyanotic but …" I moved closer to Jim again, wondering what "cyanotic" meant. Figured it's not good to be cyanotic. But not bad that he isn't, right? I leaned awkwardly into him, trying for an embrace, murmuring inane reassurances, glancing at the red poinsettia next to him, yearning for cheer from it. Our old dog Hope sat attentively to one side, no doubt wondering when Jim was going to spring from his chair for her morning walk.

But now he was suddenly struggling, gripping the arms of the chair, trying to lift himself and failing, his breath coming in short, rasping heaves, and the panic was deep in his eyes and my own anxiety was bubbling up like bile and I could no longer pretend calm and we were alone together in a small boat in a storm and sinking and it was a moment before I realized that Donna had opened the front door and the living room was suddenly filled with fire-fighters and then they stepped aside for two para-medics, both of them swift and practised and all of them talking in those loud, steady voices that try to penetrate the haze of terror and they started with "Sir?" and then "Mr. O'Neill?" and then "Jim?" and they urged him to blow into a paper bag to ease his growing panic but he couldn't seem to summon any breath and then there was an oxygen tank beside him and then a mask over his face but that didn't seem to relax him at all and then he was on a stretcher and out the door and down the familiar front walk and into an ambulance with flashing lights and quickly gone away, this man whom I have loved for thirty years.

DONNA AND I followed in her car, both of us silent after sharing a tight chuckle over the realization that we had become ambulance chasers. I was grateful for her company on this first trip to any hospital in decades. She knew the way.

Trillium Health Centre is about twenty minutes west of us, an efficient drive between tidy suburban houses and scraps of old farm orchards along a road grandly named The Queensway, with a meridian that doubles as a hydro corridor. Its towers marched alongside us for a while and then suddenly veered into a field as though they had important business somewhere else. We passed front doors with candy canes and Santa Clauses and wreaths tacked to them and others that were smoothly wrapped and ribboned in bright green and silver foil like gifts, all the variations on the seasonal decorating clichés — including those grotesque hanging icicle lights that were popular that year — and I remembered that it was December 23 and thought about being startled awake four nights earlier to hear Jim retching loudly in the bathroom, a sound so uncommon in our home that I jumped out of bed, only to hear him murmur "That's better" before he crawled back into bed and fell asleep again.

A large sign announced the hospital Emergency entrance. Donna dropped me there and left to park.

Like Emergency waiting rooms everywhere, this one was a national snapshot: the very young, the very old, the not one or the other, the cranky, the passive, the annoyed, the anxious. Hard airport-style seats, welded together. Honking, sneezing, coughing. The occasional groan. A towel wrapped around an arm, the blood from a wound seeping through. Hopeful glances any time a staff member bustled past. Ominous belches, and then vomiting from the old man in the next seat. A plastic container swiftly provided. The sign-in at the admitting desk. The moment I feared.

An admissions clerk with fingers poised over a keyboard looked up and rattled efficiently through the patient's name/ address/date of birth/health card protocol. "Next of kin?"

Ah, so this is when they get you. This is when all the old horror stories about same-sex partners come back to bite and rip, from the days when AIDS was still green and hospital authorities coldly shunned any inquiries not validated by blood or marriage. This is the moment when intimacy can no longer hide from bureaucracy, when it is finally time to speak the truth out loud to a stranger who sits at a desk, a barrier between you and the person you care most about. Jim was somewhere behind her in that maze of cubicles, suffering and confused.

"I am."

"Relationship?"

"Partner."

"Name, address and phone number?" Same address. Same phone number.

It was over that quickly. No pause, no challenge, no judgement, no dismissal. Not even the subtle drop in social temperature that only minorities can sense, that faint but unmistakable shift in tone that signals a step back into the safe zone of formality. Not this time. Just the rapid clatter of a keyboard, a pleasant but harried person routinely filling blanks on a form, stitching together some sketchy information for medical staff about a patient in crisis. Otherwise-healthy 57-year-old male, non-smoker, regular exercise, good diet, stable home environment, reported to have had the flu ("Are you sure it was the Norwalk virus?"), hard to be sure but he seemed to have all the symptoms and it was never officially confirmed because victims were urged to stay away from hospitals and doctors to prevent the spread of something that would resolve on its own anyway, advice apparently ignored by many of the people hacking behind me in the waiting room. "Have a seat," the clerk said. "You can see him in a few minutes. Next?"

DONNA AND I waited more than an hour, our effort at conversation finally eroding into desultory monosyllables.

"Time?"

"Ten past. Coke?"

"No, thanks. Should be soon."

"Should be."

Then the clerk called "O'Neill?" and we were led by a nurse down a short hallway into the Emergency Ward itself. Jim was lying in a cramped cubicle with flimsy curtains drawn around it and he had wet himself, a large spreading stain on his sweatpants. But he seemed unaware of the stain and its smell, and I was grateful that humiliation had not been added to his discomfort. Donna and I stood on each side of his bed. I think he knew who I was, but he had an oxygen mask on his face and I couldn't understand the faint bleats that emerged from behind it. He shifted jerkily on the bed and I realized he was trying to escape but had no energy for it. I held his hand, told him I loved him and that he was in the best place and that everything was going to be okay and not believing any of it except the love part.

But I could not be still and wait. I had to move, feeling like a street rat I once watched that ran to a fragment of pizza in the gutter and then away and then returned, again and again, feeling those clashing impulses now, to stay and to flee, drawn to him but repelled by him, by his menacing descent, back and forth, from the waiting room to the coffee shop to his bed and around the track again, resting nowhere for more than a few seconds.

Once, I heard a voice at the entrance to his cubicle: "I like your hat." Some tweedy thing with a peak that I'd forgotten I was still wearing. A friendly nurse named Mary, the keeper of information about Jim's diagnostic progress, smiled at me. "Is it Irish?" Later, she would tell Donna she has a gay brother.

I nabbed a young doctor hurrying past Jim's cubicle and asked the obvious. "Don't know yet," he said. "We know he's got severe pneumonia and that both lungs are involved. We can't stabilize him. We've got a call upstairs for a consult. Should be here any minute. Excuse me." He was gone.

Any minute became minutes became hours. Goddamn doctors. All the same. Probably on a golf course somewhere nearby, ignoring his pager while he lines up a putt. A bizarre thought for a cold winter day, but there it was. Mary paged him again.

BILL MCMULLEN finally arrived in Emergency two hours later, a compact doctor with silver hair and a trimmed beard. Something to do with internal medicine. I wasn't sure. He sat down at a nearby desk, taking notes from a computer screen, and then rose to assess Jim. I intercepted, introducing myself, and he dodged past me, drawing the cubicle curtain closed with a swoop.

"He's a tight one," observed Donna, wise to the political landscape of hospitals after thirty-two years as a nurse. We lingered outside the curtain. McMullen opened it a few minutes later and headed briskly for the desk again. He picked up a phone.

I intercepted again and pressed, too anxious and belligerent to back down: "What's going on? What's wrong with him?" McMullen finally focused on me and paused before responding. "He's very sick. We have to get him up to Intensive Care. I'm trying to arrange for a transfer." He punched some buttons, cradled the phone receiver on his shoulder and turned away from me.

Much later I would learn that McMullen is a very good doctor and a genuinely nice human being whose dry sense of humour had fled him that day. Jim was slipping fast and he knew it and there wasn't a damn thing he could do without quick, serious help and, sorry, I can't care who you are to him right now because you're in the way so could you please just stand over there while we try everything we've got to save him.

Our paths would cross again, and we would become cautious allies in Jim's care. But I still don't know if McMullen plays golf. I never asked.

IT WAS SIX O'CLOCK, eight hours after I had watched Jim leave home on a gurney.

Donna and I could only assume it was dark outside by now. Two hours before, we had begun our vigil on a tired couch in a windowless family lounge down the hall from the Intensive Care Unit that now held him. A TV flickered silently from its perch high on a wall, watched by a man in a baseball cap who nodded to us when he entered. He slumped in a chair, the beak of his cap pushed back over his head, entranced by the rapid movements of cartoon figures on the screen. The three of us were the only people in the large room.

Every few minutes, I would rise and call the nursing station from a desk inside the waiting-room entrance, a desk with a sign that announced a volunteer was sometimes on duty there and that visitors were required to call the nursing station before entering the ICU. "Can we see him?" Not yet. They're still settling him in. We'll let you know.

Finally, we were invited to a tiny room tucked around the corner from the Intensive Care desk, Donna and I and Neil Antman, and I knew it was an island of privacy for the bad-news chats. Antman is an intensivist, a freshly-minted word that describes a physician whose speciality is caring for the critically ill. He has a friendly, open face with the demeanour of a peewee hockey coach whose team might not make the finals but you've gotta give it all you've got anyway, boys. He was hunched forward, sombre, seeking language that walked carefully around hard truth. "I have to tell you," he said, "that Mr. O'Neill is gravely ill. His prognosis is not good. His lungs are in failure and his organs are starting to shut down. At the moment, he needs full life support." He sighed. "I'm sorry." Donna and I looked at each other. I could not accept what Antman said. It was all too quick, like a sudden fall down a deep hole. "I want to see him," I said.

Antman gave me a room number and directed me around the corner. Donna stayed behind, waiting at the nursing station.

At first, I thought I had stumbled into the wrong room and I started to back out, ready to apologize for intruding. This wasn't Jim. This couldn't be the active, bright, funny, generous man I live with. Not that distorted face, not what I can see of it in the dim light, past all the monitors and the respirator and the staff ringed around him like sentries. It can't be Jim. Jim wears glasses. This man has no glasses. I've made a mistake.

I wavered, then moved closer to the bed, peering. Yes, this was Jim. This was Jim, dying, his face looking strange and deformed. Staff had drugged him into unconsciousness. "We need to control his body's shutdown so that the respirator can keep doing its work," a nurse explained. "We need to ease the strain on the rest of his organs. We don't want him to crash." She registered my shock. "Don't be alarmed. It's standard procedure," she said.

Through the evening, his blood pressure dropped some more and his temperature jumped and his heart rate faltered and his kidneys and liver continued to fail and his lungs were fully dependent on the respirator for oxygen.

Around 10:30 p.m., a nurse suggested that family be notified and I took that to mean that the end could be close. Or maybe it didn't. I was learning very quickly that health care professionals often hedge. They find shelter in probabilities and conditional responses. No one could tell me with any certainty what would happen next. But his brother Al and his two sisters, Mary and Kathy, would want to know what I knew, as tenuous as it was.

I had called Mary much earlier in the day and told her that Jim was at Trillium Emergency. She and her husband John live in Oshawa, about an hour from Toronto.

"Good," she said.

"Good?"

"I only mean good that he's finally being looked after. I didn't like the sound of his cough when I called yesterday. I told him he should see a doctor. He said he was getting better, remember?" I remembered.

I had also called her from the hospital several times since, keeping her apprised, telling her about the long wait for attention in Emergency and about McMullen's vague responses and then about the decision to transfer him to ICU.

I called her again now and asked her to pass the word about his scary continuing decline to Al and Kathy, both even further than Mary, both of them hours away. "I've stayed in touch with Al and Kathy," she said. "Everyone's coming in. We'll all be there."

What now? Wait for them? Nah, I'll go home and feed and walk the dog. Take a short break. See what happens. Maybe be back by the time they arrive. Donna dropped me at the front door. I fed the dog, then called the ICU nursing station.

"How's he doing?"

"About the same. No improvement."

"Should I come back right now?"

"That has to be your decision."

"Well, how bad is he, compared to earlier?"

"He's not doing well."

"Should I come?"

"That has to be your decision."

It had been more than twelve hours since the ambulance had taken him from here and I could not look at the chair where he had sat that morning. The day's events and their sequence and the staff responses were all starting to blur. I hung up and tried to organize my confusion into imaginary Post-It notes. What they mean? Go or stay? He dying right now? Call Donna. She nurse, she know. Called Donna: what they mean? This some kind of code? Donna not sure.

Gotta think about this. Walk dog. Bring poop bag. 1) leash dog, 2) go outside. Lock door. Cold night. Careful: Ice.

At the rate my mental processes were racing I would soon be communicating in clicks.

Hope and I were halfway down the front walk before I

realized Donna's car was at the curb. She was standing at the driver's door and spoke over the car's hood in a low voice but I could hear her without effort on the deserted winter street. "I've been thinking. They can't come right out and say it because the roads aren't good — they can't advise you to take risks. But I believe they're suggesting you should come. Soon as Hope does her business I'll take you there."

Back at the hospital, Jim's slide continued. A solemn watchfulness had set in around him, with nurses drifting from machine to machine to chart his descent. Mary and John arrived around midnight, followed around 1 a.m. by Kathy, his other sister from Trenton and one of her daughters, and then by Al and Shirley, his brother and sister-in-law from Peterborough. They all looked dazed and unkempt, as though they had dressed in haste, and they bent over his bed and shook their heads. Shirley turned to me. "I can't believe it's only nine days since you had us all for dinner," she said. "I can't believe he's so different."

Knowing they would stay, I asked Donna to take me home again around two, tried to nap, called the hospital instead, heard nothing new, called Donna and told her there was nothing new and then returned to Trillium an hour later, this time on my own but still drawn and repelled, coming and going from it, tasting its edges and then retreating. Jim's brother and sisters were taking turns by his bed.

Finally, we all huddled together in the family lounge, too stunned and tired to say much. A woman slept on a nearby couch, tucked in with pillow and blanket. What was spoken: "He's a fighter." What was unspoken: "He won't make it through the night."

But he did, surprising everyone. Around 4:30, the nurses placed something called a cold blanket under him. It's normally used for stroke victims to slow blood flow to the brain. In Jim's case, a nurse made it clear it was a last-ditch effort to lower his temperature from its stubborn hold on 104 degrees. The strategy seemed to work and his temperature drifted down slightly. Still elevated, but something had been reversed and we saw it as reason to hope. He wasn't getting better, not at all, but he had stopped getting worse. For now, at least. For the first time, it was finally possible to feel some relief.

We all dispersed at 6 a.m., Jim's family facing long drives but wanting the comfort of their own beds. I went home to the comfort of denial.

HADN'T SLEPT. Hadn't really tried. It was Christmas Eve, after all, and I was wide awake and there was a lot to do so why the hell wasn't anything but doughnut shops and convenience stores open at 6:30 a.m., what with all this bombast about a global economy and business at full throttle somewhere else in this 24/7 world, with last minute shopping and banking to do and cards still to mail but no stamps — shit! — and the house to clean before the final decorations went up. They would be late going up, but what the hell. I paced and muttered, aware he had been in hospital for twenty-four hours, certain they would release him today. He was a healthy guy. He would be right out the other side of this in no time. I wanted to be ready for back to normal.

So that morning I did all the things of a normal day but with obstreperous intensity. Wished the bank teller a Merry Christmas, too loudly, too heartily. Drove too frantically. Walked too briskly. Bought the stamps and flung the Christmas cards into a mail box. Everything too this, too that. Pushed through a list of mundane chores, all exalted to imperatives, all the while convinced I could outrun my foreboding. Until, finally, I was home again and the milk was in the fridge and the bread was put away and the two boxes of flowers from solicitous neighbours were stuffed temporarily into a pasta cooker and a juice jug because Jim would know how to coordinate them into the right vases and Hope was fed and I could now slouch at the dining room table to gaze across to where he always sat for our morning coffee and for all the daily meals that followed it like welcome punctuation points.

I looked through the air that had replaced him, looked at a small painting now revealed on the wall behind his empty chair, knew in that moment that I was witnessing our dismemberment. I could hear the old clock ticking in the next room and the dog snoring softly beneath the table, found no solace in those familiar sounds, and I wept.

TWO

No change: a phrase that can either calm or chill on the whirl between hope and dismay. It rides on inflection, on emphasis, and it requires alertness in the listener to mine its implications because I had already learned that nothing explicit is ever conveyed in a phone call to an ICU nursing station. No change: had his decline been halted? Did that mean he was stable? No change: was he continuing to weaken? I knew from the nurse's regretful tone when I phoned after vigorous nose-blowing and throat-clearing that the news was not good. "No change." She sounded discouraged.

The cold blanket tucked under him had lowered his temperature for only a few hours. Now it was climbing dangerously again, and he remained unconscious.

All through the long Christmas Eve afternoon, I watched nurses glance at monitors that confirmed things they already knew, make notes, consult a computer in his room and key in unexplained entries, smile at family in that distracted way of the tired and resigned, speak in do-not-disturb tones reserved for the sleeping.

He can't hear us. You know he can't hear us. Why is everyone whispering?

Once in a while, a respiratory technician would try easing Jim's oxygen support back from 100 per cent to 90 per cent, then quickly return when the ventilator began to beep and then it would be dialled up to, maybe, 95 per cent, let's try that, and the respirologist would be back in minutes because the machine had beeped again so let's see how he does at 96 or 97 per cent and finally there would be a huddled conversation between nurse and respirologist, and the oxygen setting would be pushed to 100 per cent support again.

I had already begun to realize that the alarm signals from hospital monitors are merry little chimes, electronic ding-dongs not unlike those benevolent daily reminders that the microwave has thawed the TV dinner or the car seat belt hasn't been fastened. Even a Code Blue call, the universal and imperative hospital summons to a serious medical emergency, is voiced through the PA system with the kind of tranquil detachment normally reserved for flight announcements. So at first it was startling to watch staff respond to friendly chirps like someone had crept up behind them with a prod, as they did every time Jim's heart rate faltered or his blood pressure dropped. It seems no noise is good noise.

Mary and John and Al and Shirley and Kathy had arrived again, all of them showing their lack of sleep, their conversation tight and forced. Mary wore a veneer of self-control and it cracked once, when she leaned into me in tears. Kathy stood back, wringing her hands, taking her reaction cues from her older siblings. All of us could only gape at Jim and fret, taking turns on the path back and forth from the waiting room. By now his chest was tapped with three tubes and a nurse explained they were necessary to drain fluid from his lungs. Always slight, he had swelled to a size that might have cheered him through his recent weight-lifting campaign to add muscle and bulk. But his face, hands and feet were also bloated, the result of fluid leaking into his body from a tear in one lung. "He looks like the Michelin Man," said Al, who can sometimes be flippant, even in a crisis, and I thought he was reaching for levity with the comment, then realized that his face remained solemn as he stared at Jim and I agreed with him, silently wondering if one day we would laugh about this resemblance to a tire icon.

I saw Neil Antman behind the large nursing station and pursued him, stalking for answers. "I'm not looking after Mr. O'Neill today," he said over his shoulder on his way to another patient. "If you have any questions, ask for Dr. Murthy."

My first impression of Anant Murthy was that he was quick, smart, confident and glib. He had very white teeth and a cheery smile and both assets were in play when he told me, almost breezy and offhand in manner, that all their efforts to save Jim were failing. I wanted to slug him. I watched him look down and then up and then away as he spoke, never meeting my eyes, and it was a minute or two before I realized how profoundly uncomfortable he was with the task of conveying unpleasant information, that he seemed incapable of assuming the sombre demeanour expected of him. He did not dodge the truth. Nor did he cloak himself in solemn platitudes. He simply presented bad news with a smile, and the incongruity was unsettling. I had some sympathy for his discomfort, suspected his smile was an uncontrollable impulse, even wished a speedy end to the conversation for his sake. I still wanted to slug him anyway.

In an effort to be ready for the worst, I began to make silent plans for Jim's funeral and burial, knowing that he would want to join his parents in the little country cemetery that rolled gracefully down the road from the yellow-brick ancestral church. Familiar names on all the tombstones, anchoring him to his roots in our early autumn strolls together while the wind played with the trees and he told me the stories that stitched together into the tapestry of his past.

Al and Shirley and Kathy went home. John and Mary and I remained, sometimes all together with Jim, sometimes taking turns.

Much later that evening, a gentle ICU nurse built like a linebacker approached us and asked if we'd like him to summon a clergyman for Jim. Another hospital code, this one unpublished but obvious in its implications. His name was Mike, he said, and he presented the list of denominational options like a diffident waiter. We chose a Catholic priest from the menu.

Father McMillan ("Call me Neil.") arrived in about half an hour, an avuncular man who followed us into Jim's room and unpacked the oil and the crucifix and the prayer book, the essentials for administering Extreme Unction. Sometimes called the Last Rites. Sometimes called the last chance for lapsed Catholics to slip back into favour before dying and otherwise going immediately to hell.

Jim and I had finally turned away from a church that has no accommodation for committed gay relationships and that officially condemns homosexuality as an "intrinsic moral evil," but we both still felt its primal tug. For many former Catholics, the ache of separation from the church of their childhood never really disappears. It is the ghost in the corner.

Neil knew nothing of our struggle and his benevolent presence was welcome because it carried no baggage. Jim was only another very sick patient and he seemed unruffled by having to surrender a piece of his Christmas Eve to the crisis. Mary, John and I stood beside him. He avoided gloomy exhortations and prayed for Jim's restoration to full health, then wished us all a Merry Christmas and hurried away.

Hours later, in the middle of the night, after Mary and John had left, I stood at the hospital entrance, guilt and grief mixing with the smoke from a cigarette, defiantly abandoning my campaign to quit or at least cut down. A cleaner taking a break a few feet away tapped an ash, glanced at my own cigarette and nodded at me conspiratorially. "Feels like snow," he said. "Bet it's gonna be a white Christmas." Behind us, inside, Emergency staff chatted in small groups, likely wondering how long the waiting room would remain empty. Cars drifted by at the languid pace of the tired and the cautious. I heard a voice in my head, clearly and distinctly: "This is not his time." No shaft of light from the darkness above or rustle of angels' wings, no shimmer of reassurance and consolation overlaying the words. A dispassionate voice, almost a news reader's neutral voice, with just enough weight to present a fact without bias or colour. I glanced furtively at the hospital cleaner, still a few feet away, still smoking, still staring at the street, waited a minute for more pronouncements from the sky and when none came, turned and went back in.

"This is not his time." I carried those five words with me up the elevator and then the stairs back to ICU, back to the humming, twinkling machines, back to search staff faces for any flickers of hope. Secure in my understanding of incongruity now, one truth expressed downstairs by the voice, another expressed upstairs at his bed, no meeting of the two. I kissed him goodnight and left.

THREE

"When are you coming in? We need to talk." Anant Murthy was on the phone, pulling me out of a ragged sleep.

It was Christmas morning and it had snowed overnight, validating the hospital cleaner's conversational prediction. News about Jim had rippled up and down our quiet street, the report of both a fire truck and an ambulance too dramatic to ignore. Neighbours leaned on their shovels and chatted in small groups, occasionally glancing at our front door. Someone had shovelled the front walk, and then the long sidewalk that borders the house and leads to the driveway.

Brenda and Delia from a few doors up on the other side had paused with their dogs to talk to Firefighter Bob on the corner diagonally opposite us and from their faces I knew what they were talking about because Bob had seen the ambulance arrive and watched Jim leave in it. Jamie, Ken and Mary's son, home from school, was making snowballs across the street but stopped when he saw me lock the front door, uncertain whether to approach. He considered, then presented a card for Jim. Rob and Ellen from two doors up had a tray of food which Rob then hastily withdrew because I was leaving and he promised to deliver it later. Rob and Barb from next door volunteered to field inquiries about Jim's status, undertook to dispense regular updates to callers, sparing me the need to express awful uncertainties more than once. Ian the burly tree expert came around the corner and when he asked how Jim was doing tears came to my eyes and he then gave me a hug so ferocious that my breath released in a wailing honk. When I left for the hospital, my car had been cleared of snow and ice. All I had to do was start it and go.

"WE'VE TRIED everything and now we have no more options here." Even on Christmas Day, with a jolly seasonal banner drooping over his head at the nursing station, Murthy refused to gift-wrap reality. Annoyingly, he was still smiling.

"My gut tells me that if he stays here, he will likely die. We can't get his lungs to function. He just can't breathe on his own, and his lungs are badly damaged. He might have a chance at survival if we can get him into Mount Sinai ICU but I'm not optimistic. They're using a new respiratory procedure down there. Frankly, I've read the studies they've done about it and I'm still not convinced. You should know there's a high risk he could die in transfer, between here and there. Also, he needs dialysis because his kidneys have failed. We don't have dialysis here and Sinai does. It's a long shot but I'd still recommend it. However, the decision has to be yours."

"Take the deal." Bizarrely, all I could think of was Steven Hill, the actor who played rumpled district attorney Adam Schiff for ten years on Law & Order. Weary, morose, reconciled to imperfect justice, Schiff would often counsel his deputies to pocket their idealism in favour of compromise. "Make the call," I said to Anant Murthy. "Please find out if Sinai will take him. If he dies on the way there, I'll take responsibility." Murthy shook his head. "No, you won't," he said. "If he dies, I'll be the bad guy. That's part of my job." He was no longer smiling.

Murthy left to organize the transfer and returned a few minutes later to confirm that Mount Sinai ICU had agreed. We shook hands. I was the brave partner, stepping up to make a choice that could kill Jim, and I was a nervous but proud collaborator in his possible deliverance. Or so it appeared. But I knew even then that I was still circling, still pulled and pushed, and so I asked Murthy to lay out the either/or of it for the rest of the family, now straggling back to Trillium on highways made treacherous by more snow. On one level, I didn't want Jim's transfer to look like the unilateral decision it had been. On another, I needed to share this risk with them, needed them to feel included in this process, yes, needed their approval even though the hospital had tacitly acknowledged me as his next-of-kin with the right to a tormenting power. They could relax with our relationship at family social events but I had no way of knowing how they would react to a life-or-death decision like this. It was unfamiliar terrain for all of us.

Finally, everyone who could be present was present: Mary, accompanied not by John who had stayed behind to cook Christmas dinner and mind the grandchildren but by their sons, Rick and Dave, and Al and Shirley, and Kathy and her daughter Janice. Murthy gathered us all in an empty ICU room and we stood in a corner while he sat on the edge of the vacant bed and repeated the options. This would be the rock and that would be the hard place. I cleared my throat and announced that I supported moving Jim to Mount Sinai, even with all the risks.

There was silence for a moment. "I don't really think there's anything to discuss," said Mary, always the pragmatist. "I say we go with the only chance we've got." There were nods from Al and Kathy but they said nothing, deferring to Mary and to the doctor, apparently withholding any active support of my role. It was some time before I realized they were also deferring to me, that they had already crossed a bridge that existed only in my imagination. I felt the full weight of Al and Kathy's trust. But I was unsure of Mary and she of me, and that was clear.

Then we had to wait while they prepared Jim for transfer, not as simple as easing him onto a gurney and whisking him out the door. Instead, the nursing team had to make sure there would be no interruption to the high level of his care. He would remain on a respirator all the way, and the monitors and feeds would travel with him. Effectively, he would be in an ICU room on wheels. Normally there are two paramedics staffing an ambulance, one to drive and the other to attend the patient in back, but Murthy had astutely requested a driver, freeing both paramedics to pay complete attention to Jim. All of these arrangements took an hour and a half.

Once Jim was ready to go, Murthy suddenly asked if I wanted to ride along in the ambulance. That invitation sent me into brief private turmoil because I had imagined I could step back and hand him over, let them take him away to uncertainty, let a telephone call serve as a protective buffer from the worst possible news, even ready to suggest Al might want to go with him. I wanted to be there if he died on the way. I didn't want to be there if he died on the way. Back and forth, conflicted again, all in a few seconds. Finally, being with him won. Finally, I decided I could not be absent from any part of this harrowing journey, that I could no longer circle it, that the sickness part of our unvoiced vows was being tested, the vows we had never expressed publicly but honoured anyway, that I had signed on for all outcomes. I buckled up in the passenger seat.

The driver and I shook hands without exchanging names. As we rolled out from the hospital and south onto Hurontario, the wide street that links to the expressway that would take us downtown to Mount Sinai, he steered with one hand and punched the radio buttons with the index finger of the other, quickly sampling "Jingle Bells" and "Silent Night" before settling on a jazz station. "I'm sick of Christmas music by now," he said. I don't want carols but I don't like jazz, I thought.

It was about five o'clock and the house exteriors on either side were illuminated with splashes of alternating red and green and blue, many with the antiseptic icicle lights that hung like tentacles from roof edges. I could imagine that people inside the warm houses were now bibbing themselves for dinner, suffused in companionable satisfaction, challenged only by the limits of their appetites. He could die right now, I thought, and he was only a few feet behind me, only a formless shape.

This was a beefier ambulance than the kind that zips adroitly around, rushing people to hospital. As big as a panel truck, its heft and weight gave it a kind of hulking majesty. When it was in motion. But suddenly we stopped, right in the middle of traffic. The driver stepped on the accelerator. The ambulance's big engine revved but we didn't budge. He tried again. The ambulance appeared to rear up with each press of the gas pedal and then rest. Cars darted impatiently around us. What happens now, I wondered to myself. Will they have to call another ambulance, start all over again? Then, ludicrously: should we all get out and push?

One of the paramedics called out an inquiry from the back. The driver ignored him and scanned his instruments, fiddled a few controls. Gave a sharp tug on a lever and then quickly released it, pulled and released again. "Damn handbrake sticks," he muttered. We had been stopped for two minutes. It seemed like an hour. We moved on.

Every few minutes, I would turn, squinting through a narrow opening between the front seats to the back of the ambulance. The light was subdued, the two figures hunched over Jim shadowed and indistinguishable. "How's he doing?" Always a tolerant "he's fine, he's okay" in response. "Sorry to keep asking," I said after we'd been on the road for about twenty minutes. By now my queries had become almost a running gag. "How's he doing?" This time, there was ominous silence from the back and I feared what I would hear.

Suddenly, a hand reached through, holding a piece of paper. "Here's your Christmas card." It was a print-out of Jim's vital signs. "Take a look. He's actually doing better than he was when we left Trillium." A helpful "good!" had been scribbled in a margin above the rows of spikes.

It was snowing again so we moved cautiously along the expressway, red and white flashes from the ambulance light bar bouncing off guard-rails and other vehicles. An eerie experience, watching cars scoot aside, brief bursts of light illuminating their interiors like cameras at a press conference. Occasionally, the ambulance driver would tap his siren, a short, burping nudge for the dozy or distracted. In his place I might have been snarling by now. But always sanguine, he behaved like a benevolent parent toward aggressive drivers playing chicken with the weather and with us. "You get used to it," he said.

Forty minutes after leaving Trillium, we arrived at the Emergency entrance of a large, square presence on University Ave. I was told Mount Sinai's ICU was on the top floor of the hospital. I thanked the driver who stayed behind with the ambulance and then the two paramedics and I escorted Jim to an elevator and up eighteen floors.

I stayed by his side and merged with the large group of doctors and nurses busy uncoupling him from the mobile hardware in an ICU room, their own equipment ready to one side for the swap. Calm, efficient moves, focused completely on Jim, gathering information from the paramedics while they worked, trading clinical comments with each other. No one paid any attention to me, fretful at the perimeter. "Hi, I'm Patrick," I prattled like a Rotarian recruiting new members at a convention. "He's Jim and I'm his partner so if there's anything you need to know about him, anything I can do to help, just ask. Want me to hold that? Is he okay? The guys will tell you he did fine on the ride in. No problems, right, guys?" A tall nurse suddenly looked up and blinked at me, startled by this stranger without a uniform or a white coat. She stepped away from the bed and eased me out, drawing the curtain behind her. "I'll show you where the waiting room is," she said, suppressing a hint of annoyance. "We'll come and get you when we've settled him in."

Family had followed in several cars and I met them in the hall, told them he'd survived the journey and showed them the print-out and pointed to the encouraging "good!" and urged them all to go home and make whatever Christmas they could for children and grandchildren. I would call later, after I'd seen him. Rick, Jim's nephew, had driven my car in and told me where he had parked it. "I think you need a tune-up," he said. Everyone lingered, uncertain. "Go on," I said. "I'll be fine." They left reluctantly.

Another waiting room, this one with windows and carpet and dark, posh furniture and a very large family, the faces impressed with familiar anxiety, the low voices rough and intense. Trays of food crowded every surface. We waited, the large family and I, heads turning in unison every time someone appeared at the door. Some time later, the lead paramedic came in and shook my hand, wishing me well. "Won't be long before you can see him," he said. "We've signed off." I thanked him and he left.

An elderly woman watched him go, then turned to me and smiled. One of the big family, I thought, but on the edge of it, seated away from its anguished centre. A little bored and restless, perhaps. Ready to chat, ready to find the common ground of the distraught and the uncertain. A safe, courteous opener: "Who are you here for?"

"My partner's in there," gesturing over my shoulder. By now I was exhausted, no longer up for the pleasantries that can grease conversation between strangers bonding in a crisis.

"Your partner," she said, with mild surprise. "Doesn't he have any family? Where's his family?"

"I sent them home."

She looked shocked, then saddened. I got the sad part — who in places like this is not sad? — but the shock part took a few minutes to register. Finally, I rose and stood over her. "You thought he was my business partner, didn't you? You thought his family had abandoned him to his business partner. We're not in business. He's my life partner. We've been together for thirty years."

"Oh," she said, and I watched a small parade of conflicting reactions march quickly across her face, coming to rest on composed neutrality. "Have a cookie," she said finally, waving at a nearby table. "There's lots to go around."

FOUR

*W*hat's in a name? It's called the Intensive Care Unit at Trillium and it's called the Adult Critical Care Unit at Mount Sinai, both terms apparently inter-changeable in the language of hospitals but both places sharing the same musical hardware that sounds merriest when life is wavering. Whatever its formal title, most people call it ICU. It's where you pull up a chair and wait, quietly terrified.

Someone called my name from the waiting room doorway while I was seriously engaged in trying to figure out whether that was real leather or awfully good vinyl — do they still make Naugahyde? — on the brown wingback chair opposite, presently occupied by a large man holding a baby. On cue, I moved to another poky family consultation room like the one at Trillium, with another flabby sofa and another frowning doctor.

This one was a very young woman ("How are you? I'm Dr. Masur."), a hassled resident with sharp features now blunted by exhaustion. Mount Sinai is a teaching hospital so she was proba-bly dispatched this Christmas night by senior staff to get some practice at sharing gloomy outlooks with people other than the patient. Tidings, but not glad.

She consulted some notes, holding a clipboard in her lap. "You know how grave his condition is?" She looked up.

"Yes."

"It, uh, could go either way. You know that?"

"Yes."

"But I'm afraid it doesn't look good," she said.

I found myself trying to reassure her, us, the two of us, she and I. "He's a fighter," I said, inanely echoing the family's assertion from the previous day, and then wincing at the platitude. But it rolls so unthinkingly off the tongue at times like this, as hollow as a comment on the weather, and we take our hope from it because that's really all there is. "He's a fighter." The newspaper obituaries that cite long/brave/heroic/courageous battles with cancer/heart disease/strokes always stir me to imagine that the deceased engaged in furious hand-to-hand combat with rogue cells or faulty valves or blood-deprived brains, and finally lost. And then the terms of surrender, the dying, always gracious, always admirable, the body feebly waving a white flag at the foe within it, survivors secretly pleased that there were no messy howls of outrage at the end. We salute pugnacious valour in the dying, as long as it is tempered by good manners.

"You can see him shortly. They'll let you know," she said, and left.

So. There he lay, only twenty feet away but two walls and a corridor between us, and he was unconscious and still perhaps dying, according to the tense young doctor. A fighter? What does someone who is moribund summon for combat?

I did not fear he would deliberately submit to their pessimism. I feared he would simply retreat from all the attentive commotion, from feeling uncomfortably singled out, that he would decide that this was enough and slide away when no one was looking, in the blackest hour of the night, silently determined to exit without a fuss.

Just as he almost fled the night we met.

Tuesday, May 8, 1973, 10:30 pm. I was in a noisy gay dance bar on Toronto's Yonge Street, nursing the wounds from a failed relationship, and he was standing alone at the edge of the crowded dance floor with a mirror ball rotating above it. Wearing a turtleneck sweater and jeans. Slim, blonde, cute, self-conscious. Our eyes met and he looked away. I left the group I was with and walked over.

"Hi," I bellowed over a disco tune, summoning the aggressive joviality of the mildly drunk.

"Do I know you?" Challenging, dismissive.

I stumbled, then rallied: "No, but do you want to meet my friends back at the bar?" This was not going well but I figured adding other people might dilute the tension, might keep him engaged. He glanced at the group behind me, then at the door, ready to bolt, then paused.

Suddenly: "I guess you've noticed I have a crooked eye." I had not, so I looked and, sure enough, one hazel eye drifted askew. Why did he say that? Did he imagine I would then say goodbye and turn, relieved that a distracting physical flaw had been disclosed in advance of any potential romance? He would not know that in this moment of exposed self-deprecation he had won me with his innocence and vulnerability. He was entirely there that night, yet only a twitch away from flight. I glanced at the door. I don't want you to leave, I thought. I just want to hold you, I don't want to hold you down.

"My name is Patrick," I ventured, finally, then listened.

The clamorous disco music had stopped and Roberta Flack's "Killing Me Softly" was sliding from the large speakers. "Let's dance," I said. And while Flack's pain was strummed by cruel fingers, we circled the dance floor slowly together, graceless in our unfamiliarity with each other. I drew him so close I could feel his racing heart. You're the one, I thought. You're the one.

FIVE

ount Sinai's ICU overlooks University Avenue, facing some lumpish office buildings that obscure any view to the east. Its waiting room is on the opposite side of the building, with windows that reveal the vast flatness that is Toronto's west end, small houses and factories rolling to the horizon, church steeples and high-rise apartment buildings like pop-ups here and there. Normally the eye can take a side-trip south from the tedium for a teasing glimpse of the old Exhibition grounds and the lake to the south, but not tonight. Tonight they were masked by darkness and falling snow and I was looking at myself in the glass.

There is a small but ornate desk just inside the waiting-room door, with a phone and a little sign like the one at Trillium that suggests a hospital volunteer usually sits at it. Not tonight, of course, the dozy end of Christmas Day everywhere but here. Tonight the chair was empty and the desktop was littered with half-eaten trays of cookies and empty pop cans. A small bouquet of flowers, banned from the ICU because they might carry infection, lay discarded to one side, next to the phone. The large family was gone.

Thirty minutes after the doctor had left, promising that I could see Jim soon, the phone on the desk rang. Seven people looked at it. Seconds passed. Then a middle-aged woman left a group conversing in low murmurs and walked briskly to the desk. She was dressed in baggy sweatpants and a matching hooded top, an expedient wardrobe choice when vanity has to surrender to functionalism in a sudden crisis. She picked up the phone and scanned the room, a hint of disappointment in her voice. "Family for Mr. O'Neill? They say you can go in now."

There were some twists and turns to the going in: a right, then a left, then a mandatory pause to wash hands, then through the swinging doors, then a left past the large nursing station and then a left turn one final time to stand hesitantly at the foot of his bed. Behind me, I could hear a device somewhere next to a bed bleating an insipid version of the Avon ding-dong chime, an obvious call of distress to staff, to judge from the traffic now hustling in its direction. Another mechanical summons, but not to Jim's cubicle. The noise from his cubicle was different, a new one, something huffing — no, more like panting — sounding like a large dog after a long run.

He was still unconscious, still unrecognizable, now sprouting eight tubes from various parts of his body: his chest (several there), his back, his stomach, his groin, his mouth. If you were a horse, your ancestors would have taken pity and shot you by now, I thought.

He's from farmers, both sides, all the way back. Tough Catholics who fled Ireland in the early 19th century to trade one harsh life for another. They settled around Lindsay in southern Ontario, staked land, mixed dairy with crops, courted at church suppers, raised large families, made a little money, died at home and were

laid gently into the same earth that was caked under their finger-
nails. His mother died only weeks before her 100th birthday,
wanting to mark a century but failing, and she remembered a ride
in Lindsay's first automobile, telling the story often.

She marvelled at it. She would also have marvelled at this,
a blocky gizmo no larger than a bathroom sink chuffing at his
bedside with perky determination, his chest shuddering in synco-
pation with the rapid hat-hat-hat sound it made. The largest of
the tubes snaked from it and disappeared into his mouth and
down his throat, held in place by tape criss-crossing his face.
In this windowless cubicle with one blue wall and yellow curtains
on the other three sides, with doctors and nurses standing in
solemn vigil, he seemed to be trying to suppress a bout of chuck-
ling. His chest shook as though he and his agitated mechanical
companion were sharing some secret entertainment. At another
time, he would have covered his mouth, his eyes squinting in glee.

But this puffing apparatus with the dials and gauges was why
Murthy had proposed his risky transfer from Trillium to Mount
Sinai. It was a desperate shot at rescuing his lungs from permanent failure. We were betting his life on an experiment and my
own breath came in short gasps as I watched him.

BREATHING IS right up there on a long list of things most
people take for granted, an unconsidered act as natural and
effortless as blinking. So the body gets a nasty surprise when it
suddenly has to fight for air, and the lungs can provide a stunning
example of the domino effect. When they fail, the organs topple
one by one.

Two things are supposed to occur in normal breathing: air

is taken in by the lungs (that's called ventilation) and carbon dioxide is then replaced by oxygen (that's called respiration). Good stuff in, bad stuff out. That's what the medical profession calls successful gas exchange. That's what happens when everything is working right, when the body is able to use oxygen to keep crucial systems and organs clean and functioning.

But when breathing is severely impaired by disease or injury, most hospitals use mechanical ventilators to supply auxiliary oxygen, inflating the lungs like balloons and then allowing them to relax naturally. Most patients who don't have chronic breathing problems only need oxygen assistance for a short time before their lungs kick in again and take over the task of normal breathing. In most cases it works. In Jim's case it didn't.

With the proliferation of computers, respiratory technology has advanced a lot in the last twenty years. Now mechanical ventilators can be programmed and tweaked to provide a full range of support, from gentle supplementary breathing assistance to complete oxygen reinforcement, depending on what the patient needs. That's the good news.

The not-so-good news is that studies prove the pressure from mechanical ventilation can sometimes cause further damage to lungs that have begun to lose their elasticity, and even hasten the decline of other organs. That was already happening to Jim.

It's a Catch-22: ease off the pressure from a mechanical ventilator and the patient needing support could stop breathing. Keep the pressure up and the lungs will likely worsen if they're already stiffened or torn by disease. Jim needed full support. He couldn't breathe on his own, one attempt failing after another. In clinical terms, he wasn't oxygenating. In lay terms, he was suffocating. The respirator supplying essential oxygen was slowly killing him. Anant Murthy knew this. That's why he advocated the transfer to Mount Sinai.

But Murthy's skepticism was understandable. The medical procedure that might save Jim's life was only a few years old and it was still considered investigatory.

Appropriately, it was hatched in a neonatal incubator.

In 1972, Toronto respirologist Dr. Charles Bryan was trying to figure out how to treat premature newborns whose lungs were too underdeveloped to function correctly. Preemies often lack surfactant, a naturally occurring substance that keeps the lungs from collapsing, and doctors traditionally could only hope their little patients would survive long enough to trigger production of it on their own. It was often a case of wait and see.

On a separate research track, Bryan had been using high-frequency oscillators to measure the effects of muscle relaxants on the lungs. The two tracks began to merge. He started to wonder if oscillators could also play a role in providing oxygen to infants whose fragile lungs had difficulty tolerating the aggression of conventional respirators. Instead of introducing large volumes of air, his method would initially inflate the lungs to an optimal level, hold them open and then deliver oxygen in very rapid but gentle pulses. The idea was to achieve efficient gas exchange without unduly stressing the lungs by cycling them through a perilous expand/contract loop.

Years of trials followed and by the late 1980s High Frequency Oscillatory Ventilation (HFOV) was an accepted rescue option in neonatal Intensive Care Units around the world.

One for the babies, but grownups had to wait. HFOV trials with adults suffering serious lung disease for whom conventional ventilation has failed only began in the mid-1990s and they will likely continue for years. Mount Sinai's Critical Care Unit was among the first facilities in the world to use HFOV with adults and it's had some success, but evidence that it actually works is still largely anecdotal. All that is contended is that HFOV theoretically does no more harm than conventional respirators, marginal consolation as I watched Jim's chest flutter with 300 high-frequency pulses of oxygen a minute delivered to his lungs by the noisy machine at his bedside.

Now step aside from hypothesis for reality, for the part the textbooks never prepare you for. Learn that anything can happen and fear that it will. Witness the ancient truth of someone actually dying because their lungs just don't function anymore. Dying not suddenly or fiercely but slowly, like an evaporating stain on white sheets in a cubicle on Christmas Day.

SIX

It was Boxing Day everywhere else, the streets around the hospital choked with bargain hunters. But in ICU, a place that knows no time or occasion that is not its own, it was just another Thursday. The unit thrummed with energy and purpose. Jim was the same, a night older. The HFOV wasn't changing anything.

Two Christmas dinners from kind neighbours — "You have to eat. There's extra dressing and cranberries." — had arrived the night before when I finally went home, and I picked at them lethargically, muttering reassurances at a confused old dog. I burped once or twice afterwards, glancing nervously around at the shadows, and thought of Scrooge and his dismissal of Marley's ghost: "You may be an undigested bit of beef, a blot of mustard. There's more of gravy than the grave about you, whatever you are."

I burped again now, gently, discreetly, this cold morning. Jim's niece Janice was with me as yet another young doctor, this one named Needham, faced us in the small room off the family lounge, he in a chair, hunkered forward with a notepad, we on an old squishy couch, squirming and tense. Like the others, he was trying to be very clear about the prospects for Jim's survival, expressed this time in numbers. As in, "There is still a high probability he will die. You're aware of the survival stats on people who contract ARDS?" It sounded like cards. Or AIDS.

"Stats on what?" I asked, befuddled.

"ARDS," he repeated. "Acute respiratory distress syndrome. Your partner is being treated for ARDS." Then he paused at our puzzled reaction. "You didn't know that, did you? No one told you he has ARDS."

Janice and I looked at each other. She shrugged.

"No," I said, and for the first time I realized no one had ever given any of us a precise diagnosis of Jim's illness.

We knew the *what* of his deadly condition but not the *why*. We knew that he was in respiratory failure and that his organs were quitting one by one as a result, sending his body into chaotic descent. That, we understood. But all of it caused by double pneumonia, as the first resident who saw him in Emergency concluded? People get pneumonia every day. Some of them even walk around with it, feeling lousy but otherwise leading normal lives. It is often called the old person's friend, taking the frail and the compromised into a welcoming sleep. Jim was neither old nor frail.

We had seen the trees. No one had talked about the forest. We had not asked.

Jim was not in cardiac arrest when he was admitted to Trillium Emergency so the doctors reasoned that his severe and sudden respiratory failure was obviously due to some other cause. But all they knew for certain about his condition that first morning was that both lungs were highly inflamed, resulting in a loss of their function and therefore impeding essential transport of oxygen to the blood. What they also soon determined, however, was that his kind of pneumonia was pneumococcal, caused by an aggressive infection and not a virus. Worse, the infection was spreading rapidly from his lungs and had begun to assault his entire body, like rioting prisoners on a rampage. When an infection overwhelms the body like that, it's called sepsis, and it's deadly. It travels rapidly everywhere, even into the bloodstream. It was outpacing their effort to save him.

When modern medicine has to step back and scratch its head because a patient's illness defies tidy labelling, its practitioners reach for the handy word "syndrome." It becomes a versatile basket for signs and symptoms occurring together and pointing to an underlying disease. The young doctor assumed we knew Jim had acute respiratory distress syndrome (ARDS). He was wrong.

Unlike severe acute respiratory syndrome (SARS), ARDS is not infectious. Unlike SARS, its mortality rate is high. Although it was first described in 1967, no effective therapy yet exists to treat the disease. There are no wonder drugs or miracle cures. ARDS often strikes the vulnerable, like newborn infants, or the traumatized, like heart surgery patients or combat casualties, but there are no typical cases.

Further, it's a hard one to nail because there are a dozen probable causes. In Jim's case, doctors could only speculate. He had either inhaled bacteria-laden vomit into his lungs (some varieties of flu typically launch with unexpected and aggressive vomiting) or his immune system had been hammered by the flu itself and the bacterial army lurking in his system, the bacteria present but normally dormant in every human body, said, yippee, now's our chance. First, we take the lungs.

Doctors will usually order oxygen support to help ARDS patients breathe until their lungs start to heal by themselves.

That's the theory. That's the hope. That's when the mighty 21st century health care system is reduced to crossing its fingers. That's why Jim was induced by drugs into a coma and intentionally paralyzed. The idea was to prevent him from reflexively fighting the respirator, a natural response to discomfort, and to make sure all available oxygen went to critical organs. But even choosing the correct combination of antibiotics to treat his infection was tricky, they admitted. Dealing with ARDS gives fresh meaning to the adage that medicine is often only guesswork.

There are no national walks or tag days for ARDS — "Guess it's just not sexy enough," said one respirologist — and I'd never even heard of it before this crisis. There are no statistics available for Canada but I've been told that more than 150,000 cases are reported in the U.S. every year. That's about three times the rate for AIDS (another syndrome) or for Parkinson's Disease. Its most famous casualty is the Muppets' Jim Henson who died in 1990. It is an equal-opportunity killer that apparently cannot be predicted or prevented and it can strike anyone of any age at any time. One ICU doctor shook his head sadly at the memory of a healthy and athletic eighteen-year-old girl who was admitted with ARDS. She was dead a week later. Until recent years, about seventy per cent of ARDS patients died. That's down to about fifty per cent now, at least dividing the odds, with swifter diagnosis and better oxygen-support techniques sharing credit for the improvement in survival rates.

It was clear from doctors that Jim was tilting to the wrong side of the ARDS statistical divide. This was a hell of a way to meet a new acronym.

At that moment in the cramped room with Janice and the doctor, I had no interest in ARDS, but Janice is smart and curious so she asked him how to find out more. He mentioned a couple of websites and she noted their addresses. I didn't care right then about any mouse-clicks to enlightenment and paid little attention. I only wanted to know whether Dr. Needham would be looking after Jim.

It was suddenly very important to know names, even only first names, to identify the population between Jim and me, those aliens with the mysterious skills who might actually stretch and connect with us personally if we weren't merely patient and family but, instead, Jim and Patrick, those gay guys who have been together forever, and isn't that amazing. Using everything to get attention. Trying to make a we out of this, not a them and an us, so that maybe the odds could be tipped by the triumphant weight of community. An act of desperate faith. Enlisting them, one by one. That was the first impulse, the first imperative, to cultivate this alliance, although I did not know why then. Then, it was only about fleeing the bleakness of the crisis by attaching faces and names to the strangers who can fix people.

"So, are you the one's going to be looking after Jim, Dr. Needham?" I asked.

"Actually, I'm transferring out of here to another hospital. Today's my last day." He gave an apologetic frown, wished us good luck and left.

SEVEN

*C*harlotte was the principal nurse assigned to Jim that day, watching him all the time, and she said she would only be with him for the day, before rotating out. Seen-it-all Charlotte, serenely experienced, a veteran who said she worked now only when she felt like it or when she was really pressed by the unit brass to fill in. She preferred retirement. "These younger ones," she said, looking around at her colleagues. "I don't know how they do it, how they keep up the pace." As she did once, too, but not envying them now. Not wanting it anymore, this life as stressed and corrosive as pro football.

Without removing my coat, I sat on a steno chair beside her, a chair temporarily vacated by another nurse, and was suddenly aware of the noise that wrapped the unit, the constant overlay of machines and voices that never receded. It was like being in a small factory and the low din partnered with a repeating slide-show as time passed: Charlotte's peaceful face, the chart on her tiny desk a few feet from the foot of Jim's bed, the breathing apparatus, his rigid form in the bed, his bloated hands, the nursing station behind us with staff grouped in conversation about other patients, the lights on the monitors, the ceiling tiled with soiled squares,

Charlotte squinting to check a numerical read-out, Charlotte annotating his chart, Charlotte turning to me.

"You might want to try and get some rest," she said. "Whatever happens, you'll need all you have for this."

He remained unconscious, lost to me and to himself. But each time could be the last, each goodbye could be final, so I moved to his bedside and waited a few hours more before leaving, content only to have been there.

EIGHT

*L*ife suspends, serving only the wait. The silent telephone becomes a threat, like a loaded gun. The heart jumps every time it rings, and it rang very early next morning. "Patrick? It's Rod MacDonald at Mount Sinai."

Who? A tighter grip on the receiver. Is it over? "Yes," I said, in a low croak. Trying again, stronger this time: "Yes?"

He read my tentative acknowledgement accurately, and hurried to reassure me: "It's okay, he's stable, your friend made it through the night. I'm not calling with bad news," he said with intuitive compassion, earning my gratitude. It turned out that MacDonald was a senior respiratory therapist at Mount Sinai and he was calling to propose that Jim might be a candidate for a trial group. It wasn't MacDonald's fault that I couldn't seem to assimilate what he was saying, what the trial was all about. It had something to do with trying to figure out if mechanical ventilation can be tweaked and refined to approximate the benefits of HFOV without damaging the lungs. It sounded like he was seeking my consent to remove Jim from his HFOV machine and place him back on a conventional respirator. But hadn't he been removed from a conventional respirator in the first place because it wasn't working?

Wasn't that why he was now at Mount Sinai?

Yes, but Jim wasn't responding to HFOV as quickly as the team hoped. The trial therapy could help. Or maybe not. They were waiting before making a decision, watching Jim for their cues. He was right on the edge of being a suitable candidate for the trial. MacDonald and I talked through the risks but I was too fogged by exhaustion to understand much. I only needed to know that Jim would not be placed in serious danger. Whatever the therapy of choice, the goal was lung recruitment, a phrase I was hearing for the first time, and MacDonald patiently explained that the respiratory team's work was all about trying to bring Jim's lungs back into play, to recruit them back to normal function. He greeted every question with a compliment, like a teacher encouraging a precocious student, and I began to wonder if he was out to enthusiastically recruit more than Jim's lungs into an exploratory medical campaign. Next-of-kin was being invited to play roulette, I knew, but flattery was starting to overtake anxiety. But that's just MacDonald, I heard later, just who he is. He's often tapped for speeches and seminars, and he approaches respiratory therapy with the passion of an evangelist, eager to win converts to a full appreciation of our friends, the lungs. Gosh, those little guys — you'd be amazed at what they do. He accepted my verbal consent, giving him standby permission, but promised to have something ready for a signature anyway by the time I arrived at the hospital.

Standard ICU practice is one nurse for each patient. Today, Jim had two, Laura and Marcia. I didn't ask why. The consent form was waiting at their little desk and I picked it up to study it. Maybe I could finally grasp what was being proposed.

"Don't bother signing that," said a male voice behind me.

"We probably won't need it." I was relieved. I knew my signature would have been a frightened scrawl. I knew it would formalize permission to risk.

He was another respiratory therapist, a member of MacDonald's team. He went on to say that Jim was starting to show clinical signs of improvement and that he might not be sick enough anymore to qualify. Apparently, the HFOV was finally starting to do what it was supposed to do. I wasn't sure what it was accomplishing, baffled by the lack of any visible change in Jim and by the numbers MacDonald's colleague was throwing around, but he seemed encouraged by the assessment results. An hour later he returned to announce that it was official, that Jim was no longer a candidate for the trial.

An hour after that, Mary arrived.

"Is this the consent form? How come you haven't signed it?" She was scanning the piece of paper, still lying on the small desk but by now irrelevant and forgotten, and she waved it at me.

"No need," I said. "He won't be part of the trial. Seems he's doing too well. That's good news."

She looked alarmed. "But what happens if there's a setback, if he gets worse again? What if they suddenly decide he could be part of the trial therapy and you're not around and they don't have written consent? Why don't you sign it anyway, just in case?" It was a plea, rimmed with anger.

I explained, perhaps too loudly, too defensively, that Rod MacDonald had accepted verbal consent from me on the phone that morning and that he would have proceeded without the signature anyway, calling it only a formality. It was even less essential now. That didn't reassure Mary.

"I don't understand why you won't sign the damn thing,"

she said, her own voice rising. "It only takes a second." Laura and
Marcia continued to stare intently at Jim, ignoring us as successfully
as they could while we snapped at each other right next to them.
Mary shook her head and left to cool off in the waiting room.

Mary would have signed the consent form without blinking.
I knew that. I also knew, but suspected she did not, that she was
uncomfortable with my official next-of-kin status, with its implicit
control over her younger brother's fate, so far removed from the
superficial banter at family get-togethers when same-sex relationships were never a topic. Always hospitable, she could nod to
our intimacy from a safe distance, never extending into curiosity
about it, never having to confront its esoteric and unsettling
implications. But this was different, and it was terrifying because
it brought reality into sharp close-up. As someone who had been
a nurse, she also dreaded that the hospital would not have the
authority it officially needed to proceed if Jim suddenly deterio-
rated again, that she would lose him over the absence of a
signature. I understood all this, knew she would do anything she
could for him, grieved and suffered deeply for him, and I was irrationally angry with her anyway, and she with me. In each of us,
love and panic fought over a piece of paper.

MARY AND I had always been uneasy with each other, one
sometimes liking the other, sometimes both liking each other at
the same time, sometimes not, our varying pasts driving the tone
of our relationship. By now, she had spent more than half her life
living in the same bungalow in an Oshawa suburb, working for
many years as a nurse for a family physician while John spent
decades on the line at General Motors, both of them cherishing

moderation and predictability, both of them finally retiring on negotiated schedules.

Loud voices and emotional outbursts were tacitly discouraged in their home. They raised three children in a composed environment and could walk their street and pass houses that were comfortingly like theirs, occupied by people who thought and acted as they did, who shared their values and priorities. They sheltered themselves as well as they could from the uncontrollable chaos they knew lurked outside their tight lives, away from the organized tidiness of their tended green lawns and washed cars and all the other essential ornaments that defined appropriate behaviour.

Both of my parents were alcoholics. House moves were frequent and often sudden. I emerged with scars from an unanchored childhood and then embarked on a journalism career that bounced and wobbled capriciously, a life with unsteady changes that I knew were bewildering to Mary and John. I came out to my parents a year before I met Jim, naively expecting acceptance and enduring lamentations instead. Mary didn't know what to make of me when we met a few months after Jim and I became a couple. Her little brother appeared to be disclosing his homosexuality, and he was now publicly partnered with someone who was brash and loud and who didn't hold a steady job, in Toronto, a city she loathed — all of the package antithetical to everything she held close. I was not a warming presence in the life of someone who believed that "don't ask, don't tell" was a sensible strategy in the avoidance of potential social unpleasantness. She was courteous but reserved.

But I didn't go away, turning up with Jim for family events as the years passed, becoming a fixture in his life and then in hers and then blending with the rest of the family. Mary and I always remained cautious around each other, never venturing into any conversation that might provoke antagonism.

Because of her nursing career, she had become the family's acknowledged health authority, taking the lead when anyone got sick, passing along updates to everyone else. On a December afternoon in 1978, she had called me at home with a health update about Jim. He was in hospital for tests. I had been waiting anxiously.

"It's positive," she said.

"Good," I said, relieved to hear the result of a liver biopsy, in my medical ignorance equating positive with good news. How can positive be bad news?

"No, not good. Positive doesn't mean good. The cancer has spread to his liver and spleen. Dr. Garvey thinks he probably has about six months to live, and only if he undergoes some pretty drastic chemotherapy."

He had endured daily radiation through his Hodgkin's Disease in 1976 when we were not yet living together. "I don't know why you're so upset," a mutual friend said at the time. "You're not even living together." He seemed to have recovered, but then, two years later, a routine physical revealed some abnormalities that led to some tests that led, finally and crushingly, to Mary's phone call. We had all been in this place before.

NINE

Jim was still on HFOV and his prognosis wasn't any better, but I was puzzled by what seemed to be a small lift in his condition. After all, he hadn't made the cut. He hadn't sunk low enough to need the really experimental stuff, a trial where his legacy might be a line entry in a medical study. But what was his status? Could I take his absence from the trial group as promising news?

Later in the afternoon on advice from one of the nurses, I went off to nab a senior doctor, someone with clout who would still be there tomorrow and perhaps even next month, and found one at the nursing station. He had the build and demeanour of a brooding James Taylor.

He broke from a conversation with another doctor and looked at me expectantly. "How's Jim really doing? I'm getting mixed signals," I asked.

"Jim ...?" There was a hint of impatience.

"O'Neill, room 12."

He reached into his shirt pocket, shuffled through what looked like yellow cheat cards and paused to scan one. He replaced the cards in his pocket. "As well as can be expected," he said.

Then he turned back to his conversation, leaving me to pon-
der the mysteries of a profession that can manage to heroically
salvage human lives and then plunge into the numbing banalities
of a TV medical drama, both at the same time. As needy for words
that can buffer reality as the rest of us, I suppose, but unhelpful
and dismissive right then. This doctor's frustrating response to
my question was also surprisingly incompatible with the candour
of his ICU colleagues.

Maybe it was just another jolting reminder that the world is
moving more steadily toward expediency while embracing the
ambiguous, even in places like this where death is a brutal daily
hazard. Still, this is cheering news for obituary writers and sympathy card makers. Or for those with a fondness for euphemisms.

In the new language of solace, no longer the exclusive prop-
erty of funeral homes, most people are not permitted to simply
die. They cross or they pass away or pass on (often truncated to
just "pass") or they go to sleep in the arms of the Lord. The final
truth, dipped and frosted. Death has become a confection. That's
as well as can be expected.

ON ROUNDS the following morning, a daily ICU event at Mount
Sinai that excludes everyone who is not an insider, a senior physician chose a resident at Jim's bedside to deliver a concise summary
of his clinical status. "As well as can be expected" was not an
acceptable answer. Later, I learned what the selected resident's
response was.

"The patient presents with generalized edema, pneumotho-
rax and hypotension. There is polymyopathy and polyneuropathy.
He has a septicaemia involving the skin which has not responded

to antibiotics. His kidneys are under-functioning, requiring dialysis. Gas exchange is poor. He has profound hypoxia. He has most probably suffered a heart attack and it is our belief that appropriate testing will confirm this should he survive. There is high suspicion that he may have suffered one or several minor strokes. Again, further testing is indicated."

The silver lining? Well, the HFOV seemed to be doing some good. And his temperature had finally begun to drop. Not by much. Not even enough for mild optimism, but the first change for the better of any kind in nearly a week. This I could share with family who yearned for respite from the terror.

I sat looking at Jim and realized that even if he were to suddenly rise from unconsciousness and struggle to awareness he would see nothing. He would not see that I was there. His eyes were covered with gauze pads, placed there to compensate for moisture loss. He would be blind. See me, I prayed. See that you are not alone in this.

TEN

*A*nother day. The boy was about ten and he sat in a corner, robotically playing one of those hand-held computer games, fingers skipping nimbly through the strategies, removed from the adults around him. But tears were running down his face. He ignored them. I discreetly handed him a box of Kleenex from a nearby table and he accepted it silently, without embarrassment, without acknowledgement. He blew his nose and wiped his eyes perfunctorily and then resumed his game. His grandmother was dying across the hall. That's all I knew.

On the other side of the waiting room, four young men hovered over a middle-aged woman on a couch. She was beautiful. Impeccably and expensively groomed, she raged quietly, pain and confusion twisting an elegant, privileged face. She reminded me of tragic heroines — Euripedes' Medea somehow came to mind — and she wrapped her grief around her like a cape. Like Jim and the grandmother, her husband also lay in a cubicle across the hall. The four young men were their children. A surgeon, one of the sons told me. A surgeon who had never smoked and who was stricken with lung cancer. Where is the sense in that, the justice?

Went into cardiac arrest at Princess Margaret, the cancer hospital next door. Transferred here, doing badly. That's all I knew.

That's all anyone can ever know about anyone else in a hospital waiting room, where people twirl and sway around each other like square dancers, very careful to step lightly.

But Syd, here for the second long day in a row and therefore a veteran, wanted to know how Jim was doing. Syd who had flown back from a Florida vacation with his wife because her 85-year-old mother had suddenly collapsed, Syd who sported a fading tan and dressed like a golfer, now dropped into a deep Canadian winter while a daughter pondered her mother's imminent death. A likeable guy, obviously accustomed to resilience and action, eager to chat but starting to wilt from the corrosive wait. First names for both of us. Right now, his wife was at her mother's bedside, negotiating a comfortable end for an old woman. "She may surprise us. She may have one more round in her," he said without conviction. "So. How's he doing, your friend?"

I could say the word "better" but not believe it fully. His fourth day on HFOV and they said he continued to respond favourably, but they were doing something or other to him in there and I wasn't allowed to see him yet so I sat with the boy who was learning too soon about loss and with the inconsolable wife and the sons positioned at her side like bodyguards and with Syd, anticipating the phone call that would clear my entrance.

Then the phone call and the turns right and left, the hand washing, and the turns again — all of it by now quickly a familiar routine — and I dragged a chair close to the head of his bed, to be more alert for any hint of his return. I had to wrestle its bulk carefully past IV poles and monitoring lines and tubes and — oh, yes — the HFOV machine, gasping dutifully.

They had removed the dialysis machine because his kidneys were starting to function again and they told me there was some slight general improvement, voiced it cautiously, no false hope dispensed, and I saw none. He remained the same, still profoundly unconscious, features still puffed-up, eyes still blanked with gauze. Behind me, away from the HFOV's noisy diligence, I could hear the hum of voices and equipment, sometimes a moan from the next cubicle, and I thought about this place. It is another country, apart from others, a tiny nation with its own rituals and priorities, its borders defined not by revolution but by certainty of purpose.

As it happens, there was much bickering outside its walls that day at conference tables and in press scrums about funding shortfalls and cutbacks and a rickety health care system in desperate need of repair. In here, it seemed there was no ambivalence or political posturing. There was only the work, only this moment, right now, with every patient, no rhetoric or bombast to interrupt the smooth ticking of the machinery and the efficient partnership of skills. A kind of immunity against public swagger still prevailed here and in places like it, an unspoken disdain for the proponents of fiscal supremacy. For now at least, saving lives trumped saving money.

BACKING OUT of the parking space at the hospital an hour later, I glanced over my shoulder and saw a large white plastic bag stuffed behind the passenger seat. I had forgotten. It had been handed to me by a nurse at Trillium on Christmas Day just before Jim left and I had turned it over to Rick who would be driving my car. What they call a patient bag. What goes home with family when a patient dies or is transferred to another hospital. It held his socks, his underwear, the sweat pants with his urine stain, his T-shirt and his sweat top. No shoes. Where are his shoes? I suddenly remembered he wasn't wearing any that first morning.

At home, I removed the bag from the car and briefly considered discarding its soiled contents, tossing everything in the trash can. But I knew that would feel like I was disposing of him. So I placed the bag next to the washing machine in the basement, determined to connect with him by laundering its familiar contents, folding them neatly in readiness for him, planning a mundane distraction from our ruptured lives. But I could not go to hopefulness yet, and I left the bag where it was.

LATER THAT NIGHT, when I wasn't there, they removed Jim from the HFOV machine and held their own breath. I learned that hooking a patient up to HFOV is the easy part. But there is an optimal moment for withdrawing it. Too late and there is risk of harm. Too soon and there is risk of futility, its purpose defeated. It's all in the timing, in knowing when. "Magic is summoned, not created," said Kafka.

ELEVEN

I t is claimed that comatose people can actually hear everything we say to them — a consoling premise, but there is no
hard proof because after they awaken from a crisis, patients
usually can't remember anything that had been said. Some nurses
swear they've seen response to words — fingers lifting, eyelids
fluttering, a facial twitch, the kind of thing you miss if you glance
away. But some doctors speculate that the body protects itself
from deeper trauma, deafens itself by erasing all awareness of the
crisis, and it is left to others to tell the patient afterwards how
awful things really were. Nurses will tell you doctors don't know
everything. The smarter doctors will agree.

I figured it was worth testing the theory because this
was the Sunday between Christmas and New Year's, a drowsy
annual trough that had even lowered the tension level in the
ICU, and there was nothing better to do than to make small talk
with the nurses working with him (Laura and Marcia again that
day) and then hunker next to him for some serious chat. He
was now back on a regular respirator, and slowly beginning to
oxygenate again.

There is another theory that says that people who are very

close to death are actually presented with a choice: to proceed toward the tempting warmth of a shiny white light or to return to the hard scrabble of living. A no-brainer for some, apparently, but not yet for Jim.

I hoped he would hear me when I told him how much I loved him, that I needed him to come back, just in case he was wavering between here and the kinder light, the latter voiced loudly and firmly because he could be so far away — so loudly and firmly, in fact, that when I looked over my shoulder two visitors for the elderly woman next door and a nurse were all staring at me.

The nurse was sanguine. No doubt she had seen all kinds of outlandish behaviour by family but the visitors shuffled nervously. I didn't give a damn. Right then, I didn't care what they thought — or anyone else, for that matter. I smiled at them, then resumed my entreaties.

After a life spent looking over my shoulder, anxious for acceptance if not benediction, I had finally arrived out of terror at serene indifference to the approval of others. I didn't feel arrogant, or even defiant. In this betting on New Age earnestness, on the possibility that its proponents were right about the clear choices of the near-dead, I was also tossing an old compulsion to explain and excuse. Nearly sixty, and I realized I was finally growing up. I shouted on. "Come back!"

WELL, IT WAS soon clear it didn't suit him to come back just then — always stubborn, despite appeals — but he wasn't really going away yet either. We seemed to be at a stand-off. I went home to feed Hope and then returned that evening, feeling resolute, this time carrying something to read to him.

"The mole had been working hard all the morning, spring-cleaning his little home." So begins Kenneth Grahame's *The Wind in the Willows*, one of our favourite books. "Spring was moving in the air above and in the earth below and around him, penetrating even his dark and lowly little house with its spirit of divine discontent and longing."

Finally growing up, both of us, perhaps, but still entranced by the innocent icons of childhood and by gentle little animals who could gossip and fret and frolic. We've also owned a few clunky old wooden boats, always enjoying the tender lap of the water on the lumber of their tired hulls, and the adventurous jaunt down the river early in the book captured us forever. We were Ratty and Mole. Ratty to Mole: "Believe me, my young friend, there is nothing — absolutely nothing — half so much worth doing as simply messing about in boats."

Yes, I was reading loudly, in the reasonable belief that it's important to be heard by someone in the distance. I also wanted my voice to carry over the constant hum of machinery that surrounded us. But I also started to weep after only a few paragraphs, I don't know why, the tears dropping on the yellowed pages of the old book, shaking my head in frustration, and it was a struggle to lift the words, to put them where he could hear them. I could argue that the book somehow collects our losses, this and all the ones before, and that it summons a world we never lived in but always wanted to and that it is an anthem to unrealized dreams. I could argue all that but it doesn't matter. What mattered then, in that moment, was that my tears were intrusive and annoying, cheating any hope that he might be comforted and encouraged to come back, and I was finally forced to quit. I felt ineffectual and discouraged, as though I had somehow let him down, released his hand when I could have lifted him over the side of the boat, rescued him from his steady descent into black water and, like Ratty, jollied him into staying. Ratty would never fail Mole.

TWELVE

"You're, uh, sorry, who?" I was asking one of the residents at the nursing station for an update. He was trying to place me, trying to pair me with Jim, with room 12. Then his face lit up and he nodded. "Right, I know, I was on yesterday too. You were the guy reading to him. I heard you. In fact, we all heard you. So far today, he's stable. But just so you know, we could lose him anytime. He's not out of the woods yet, not by a long shot."

It was Monday, only a week after he had been yanked off to hospital, but it felt like a year. Donna was with me, she who had put this terrible game into play with a decisive 9-1-1 call that first morning. Like ICUs everywhere, this one limits visits to close family members and they're vigilant about that but I thought Donna had earned the right to see him. She had checked with me every day, getting restless when too many hours had passed between updates. On our way to Jim's cubicle from the waiting room, we passed a man and woman leaving the ICU. We all paused for a brief round of safe talk about the weather, an easy conversational refuge for strangers unsure of the reason for their presence in the same unsettling place. Then the man said that they had been visiting with nurses and doctors inside. "I spent two and a half weeks here," he said. "Nearly died twice. Just came back to say thanks."

Outside Jim's cubicle, I introduced Donna to Eva, one of the nurses on him that day. I had already been around enough to pick up some ICU lingo. Nurses among themselves never say they're assigned to a particular patient. They don't "work with" patients and they don't say they're responsible for so-and-so this shift. Instead, they're "on someone," useful professional shorthand that can puzzle visitors accustomed to more formal descriptives.

"This is Jim's sister, Donna," I said smoothly, and then added some credible weight: "She's a nurse too." They traded pleasantries and then Eva went off in search of supplies.

Liz appeared, the other nurse on him for the second day. He still merited the close attention of two nurses, each one spelling the other off through a shift. "This is Jim's first cousin, Donna," I said smoothly, and then added some credible weight. "She's a nurse too. Runs the day respite program at Dorothy Ley Hospice, where Jim's a volunteer." They traded pleasantries and then Liz disappeared into the adjacent cubicle.

Donna and I were standing at Jim's bedside and she was saying how well he was doing, neither of us deluding the other, when a senior nurse approached, obviously some kind of supervisor. She stopped at the foot of the bed, her arms crossed. "You're Donna?" she challenged. Donna nodded. "Which one is it? Are you the patient's cousin or his sister?" Donna looked embarrassed. I stepped forward to interject, to defend her presence, to explain why she deserved to be here even though she wasn't family, but the nurse ignored me and continued to stare at Donna. Then she suddenly relaxed. "Well," she said, "you'd better make up your mind. Please pick sister or cousin, and stay with it. Things are confusing enough around here." She smiled and left. Donna picked cousin, "I'll be cousin Donna from, uh, Windsor," but I said to hell with it and later confessed the minor transgression to staff, telling them who she was and about her vital role in this, how she had acted quickly to summon help a week before.

"She made a good call," said Eva, offering the highest tribute one nurse can give another. Donna was one of them, she had made a good call, she cared, she was welcome, sister or cousin or not.

THIRTEEN

"*H*e had cancer." First, I heard "has" and broke out in a cold sweat. Nearly twenty-five years ago this month, I remembered, and it was instantly back again, all of it, like a conga line of bogeymen returning for an encore. Undimmed by time, the sequence replayed with startling clarity: the tests, more tests, the diagnosis, the radical chemo courses that went on for months, the vomiting, the frustrating impotence as I watched him slide into weakness, the fear, always the fear of loss that finally slumped into chronic mournfulness. The dispassionate prediction by his haematologist that he had six months to live. The shame at feeling selfish, when everyone was there for him and no one for me in this pain. The lamenting that something held dear would be snatched away.

Then, the living past six months and then a year and then into years and then decades, eventually relaxing a little but with a legacy, deeply imprinted now: the uneasiness with doctors and hospitals, the overriding certainty that the news after a routine check-up would never be good. Fretting when there was an ache or the flu or even a cut that was slow to heal. Could this be a sign? Is this how it returns? He was calmer, more reasonable, through all of it.

My solution: avoid doctors. There be dragons, I was certain. It became one of his concessions to me, one of those unscripted accords that smooth every relationship. Duck-and-run had always worked. Until now.

But now, now when the past reared and snarled, it was just a new ICU doctor, glancing casually over Jim's chart for the first time, familiarizing himself with the case, making a matter-of-fact observation that required no reaction. "He had cancer." Merely some ruminative head scratching from someone fresh to Jim's condition, someone just gathering information with the curiosity of the clinician and wondering idly whether there was a link between then and now, between cancer and ARDS.

Maybe his immune system, which had been hammered by chemotherapy all those years ago, never fully recovered, making him vulnerable to infection and virus. But all of it speculation and hypothesis.

In the end, only a notation in the chart, something for them to fill a blank in a patient's history, something to remind me of the old menace woven like a repeating colour through the quilt of our relationship.

FOURTEEN

Habits can develop quickly when they're nudged by a crisis. I took to calling the nursing station to check on Jim's condition every day before I went in, a safeguard against nasty surprises. I was transferred to Eva at Jim's bedside, by now a familiar name and voice. She was excited. She had something significant to report: "He bit me."

Signs and wonders. In the 1880s, the Canadian weather service apparently took pity on remote farmers without a daily newspaper to give them a heads-up on the forecast. They were deemed not smart enough to simply look up at the sky, I guess. Someone came up with the idea of recruiting railroad trains into a campaign based on stamping out meteorological ignorance. Three different iron discs were designed to hang on the baggage cars of passenger trains, all three variations borrowed from ancient astronomical symbolism. The theory was that farmers could take pause from their weary toil in the fields, mop their brows as farmers in the classical paintings always do, watch the train rolling by and instantly know what the weather was going to be. A full moon meant fine or sunny, a crescent moon meant showers and a star meant prolonged rain or thunderstorms.

Primitive, but it worked. The future was mapped by symbols.

And a bite? Is that some kind of symbol? What does that forecast? "A bite means good news," said Eva. "I stuck my finger in his mouth and he bit it," she elaborated. I was silent. To my knowledge, Jim had never bitten anyone. Eva went on: "It's one of the few ways we have of determining various response levels in unconscious patients. It tells us Jim is starting to come around. It's primitive, but it works."

This was New Year's Eve, so there was a hint of play in the ICU. I mean a hint — no high spirits here, ever. By the time I arrived, around 9:00 p.m., Eva had more news and she was pleased. "He's bitten three of us," she announced, as though he had just delivered the perfect stool. I was number four, seconds after my coat was off. Washed my hands, stuck my index finger in his open mouth and waited. Not long. His teeth settled on my finger. Not a chomp. Not even a nibble. Just a slow, reflexive closing of his jaw. "This is good?" I asked Eva skeptically over my shoulder. "This is good," she confirmed. Recently unhooked from a state-of-the-art $50,000 breathing machine with a microchip at its core, he presented his subdued vitality with the certainty and directness of a caveman. I bite, therefore I am.

Later that night, with the lights dimmed around us and voices muted to whispers, I counted down the final seconds to midnight, to 2003, sat as close to him as I could at his bedside, holding his hand, Eva discreetly behind me at her little desk, benignly vigilant. Every time I looked over she would smile encouragingly and then resume her intense interest in the pattern of the cubicle curtain.

Jim and I had always skipped the raucous approach to midnight in all our years, thirty new years, always abandoning the parties and noise so that we could be home and alone and quiet together when each year finally turned. Always holding hands before the leap to another year. Always like this, tightly enclosed by ourselves, but not home now, now placed strangely but at least together. I held his hand and squinted at my watch in the gloom. The hour and minute hands lined up with 12. "Happy New Year," I whispered to him. "Happy New Year," I heard softly behind me, from Eva. "Happy New Year to both of you."

FIFTEEN

Like most organizations, hospitals shield themselves against intrusion with their own tribal rites and conventions, using language that can startle with its incongruity. Families and caregivers are treated as outsiders, permitted to enter for brief stays, tolerated for their eagerness and concern. While visiting, they will sometimes hear familiar words and phrases used in unfamiliar ways. I had already learned what "on Jim" meant when nurses were scheduled to look after him, but there were other pieces of hospital argot I was picking up as I went along. Some examples:

Concerning — Not "in reference to." Used within a hospital setting, the word expresses mild disquiet with a condition, read-out or test result. Typical usage: "We find his low blood pressure concerning."

Episode — "Seinfeld" had many episodes and they were fun. No one laughs at a hospital episode. Sample usage: "Today, he had an episode of seizures."

Event — Used to describe a big deal but not a good one. Heart attacks are events. Strokes are events. So are all kinds of other calamitous occurrences that result in alarmed medical staff racing around in high gear.

Evoked Potentials — Wonderful phrase, isn't it? Beckons thoughts of promise and deliverance. But it actually describes a critical test that uses electrodes to measure the electrical activity of nerves. The results are sometimes used to guide the removal of tumours around nerves. (I was sorry I asked.)

Insult — An imaginative use of the word, with an appropriate twist. Often used with an adjective to emphasize a serious point. Typical usage: "Mr. O'Neill's illness has delivered a profound insult to his body."

Outrageous — Induces vague memories of an old movie about a drag queen. In hospitals, usually employed to convey non-alarming test results. Typical usage: "His abdominal scan results are back and there's nothing outrageous."

Present — Always a verb, usually accompanied by the preposition "with." Variably "presenting" or "presented." Typical usage: "The patient presented with severe respiratory failure."

Resolved — Bears no resemblance to tenacity or to the outcome of hardy democratic debate at a meeting. Quite the opposite. Often used to describe the spontaneous and happy conclusion to a crisis that did not require aggressive intervention by healthcare staff. Typical usage: "The profuse bleeding appears to have resolved."

In this culture, as in many others, the honorific provides a respectful barrier to significant human contact. People can call each other Doctor or Mister or Miss or Nurse and retain the security of distance from each other. Hence, Jim was initially identified only as Mr. O'Neill, and I accepted the cautious formality of that until it was no longer useful.

Encouraged by his biting, the next day, New Year's Day, several nurses tried to elicit response by bellowing his name at him. "Mr. O'Neill! Can you hear me?" His eyes remained closed. One nurse leaned right over him: "Mr. O'Neill?" I tapped her lightly on the arm.

"Try Jim," I suggested. "His name is Jim. Not James, unless you're teasing him, in which case he may ignore you anyway. Jim works, most of the time."

She looked at me doubtfully but leaned into him again, her face inches from his left ear. "Jim?" Softer this time. He opened his eyes, blinked, and then closed them again. "See?" I said. "Calling him Jim works." I leaned over him. "Jim?" He ignored me. His eyes remained closed. "Sometimes," I said to the nurse.

Then I decided it was time to meet Tom, having heard much about him. "Tom? He's standing over there at the nursing station," a nurse said. "Just go introduce yourself." She pointed to a man with narrow shoulders and a friendly, open face, wearing casual clothes, smiling in conversation with colleagues.

Dr. Thomas E. Stewart is Associate Professor of Medicine and Anaesthesia at the University of Toronto and ICU Administrative Director for Mount Sinai Hospital, Toronto General Hospital, Toronto Western Hospital and Princess Margaret Hospital. All of them, all at once. He is a medical heavyweight. He lectures all over the world and is considered by his peers to be an expert in ventilation techniques used to treat respiratory diseases. He's the one Berlin or London or Chicago will call when there's a professional query about HFOV and he's as close as the investigatory protocol gets to claiming its own cheerleader. He is not grand or pretentious or bombastic. In fact, he is humble in his wonder at the way the human body heals, stepping back with a philosophical shrug when he witnesses what seems like a miraculous recovery. At work, he dresses in khakis and an open-neck shirt. He is Tom to his colleagues and co-workers. I decided to make him Tom to me as well.

Why? Complicated reasons, based on observation and response. The healthcare system does not invite intimacy. Many of its practitioners try to shy away from personal engagement, partly through conditioning by a public that holds its healers in awe and partly, I suspect, as a self-protective screen against any personal pain that might follow the loss of a patient. Many doctors and nurses see premature or unexpected death as a failure of their skills. They retreat to exaggerated courtesy, thankfully without the patronizing sneer that some cops, say, can bring to "sir." But others, usually older, actually enjoy the hierarchical nature of the system, revel in it, with its implicit power and mystery. The demeanour is usually benign, a kind of genteel condescension that comes as naturally as washing the hands after a rectal exam. But if I'm always Patrick and he's always Dr. Stewart, then our stations in this place have been set as surely as badges on shoulders or caps. As the more medically ignorant of the two, I occupy the inferior rank.

The ranks had to level. My first name? Then, your first name, please. Glad to meet you.

Truth is, I refused to be anyone's subordinate through this crisis, an early decision. The ride was hard enough. Nor did I want to pretend to know any more than I did about his clinical condition. They knew the illness, yes, but I knew Jim. I could reach back through thirty years for all the personal stuff, the foibles and behaviours and patterns, that might help complete him for them.

In a career as a journalist, I had interviewed prime ministers, movie stars, crooks and philosophers. I was seldom intimidated by fame or power because I knew I could ask smart questions and not be afraid to confess when I had not understood the answer. So I could walk into this place, happily ignorant of its customs and traditions and alien technology, and blunder through like an avid explorer because it was all fresh, all bracingly foreign. I could view a Tom Stewart with enormous respect for his skills and know that at times in my life my own had been just as honed and certain, that the creative engine had thrummed with confidence and purpose and precision.

Finally, I could look at him and be reminded that I had lived at least fifteen years longer than he had. That bought me nothing except his own courteous impulse to address someone who was clearly his senior by Mister. We got past that quickly. "It's Patrick," I said. "It's Tom," he said, and we shook hands.

And I also knew I would feel less alone in this if Jim were more than just another case with a disposable name tag. I wasn't trying to lobby for favour with his doctors and nurses. I didn't want to be their pal. In fact, I recoil from strangers who vault to the familiar, usually convinced they're trying to sell me a car or aluminium siding. I only wanted to enlist the team's full humanity to this ordeal, to remind them as persuasively as I could that the life in that bed, as tenuous and even grotesque as it then was, radiated and swirled away from them and from these borders to embrace and stir a hundred other people. And you can call him Jim.

That was the loftier motive, the one I wanted to embrace. But like many exalted enterprises, it had an embarrassing accomplice.

For the first week of his hospitalization, I had been afraid of them, all of them, their avowed commitment to healing aside. My paranoia was only now beginning to ease. But in those early days, I was secretly worried they might hurt him, could even kill him, an accident or a murder, these nameless strangers briskly moving in and out of his life, our life, and Hippocrates and the caduceus could suddenly become discussion points in a court case. A pierced line, a bent needle, a faulty valve, a clumsy turn, a missed diagnosis, even a stealthy homophobic bigot on the prowl in the darkest part of the night, driven by God to exterminate perversion. Stuff from scary books and movies and TV shows was gathering at his ICU bedside to haunt me. I was the powerless watcher who cared most about the powerless occupant. I knew this terror was not grounded in sanity. I was embarrassed, even mortified, but I also knew I had been seized by a primeval instinct to protect fiercely the one who was most precious to me. I knew that it rose from love and that fear gave it flight.

But I reasoned that they would cause him no harm, pay closer attention, link their lives to his, to ours, if I were just friendly and accommodating and chatty, in the belief that making all of the professional more personal would somehow shelter him more caringly. Ya got to go along to get along.

I was never more than a small step from dysfunction then.

So I mentally noted all their names as they rotated through his life from shift to shift, made sure they knew mine and remembered it, tried to pretend that his recovery if it happened would result from our close and collaborative partnership, and nurses who had been on him but who were now on other patients were starting to smile and wave and call me by name when I passed their cubicles on my way to his. It was we, all of us, toiling together in our prescribed roles, a smoothly ordered team, and I found sanctuary in that fanciful delusion.

"DO YOU HAVE any pictures of Jim?" Laura, his nurse again, two days later, three days into the new year, back from some time off. "He still looks pretty awful, doesn't he, even though his face isn't as puffy as it was before I left. If you had some pictures, we could tape them to the foot of the bed so everyone on staff would know what he really looks like when he's healthy and walking around." Pictures? I wasn't sure.

But a few days before he got sick, his family had gathered at our house for an early Christmas family dinner. A tense but friendly annual get-together — like all such events, bringing out the best and the worst in everyone. Kids and grandchildren were busy other places so it was grown-ups only: John and Mary, Al and Shirley and Kathy, whose husband George was absent because of the flu, and us. Hope snored on her bed, occasionally rousing to accept a compliment, then drifting back to sleep. Everyone took turns taking photos of everyone else, in groups defined by blood and marriage and conviviality. Shirley answered the call for pictures by bringing a bunch into the hospital, with one grainy close-up of Jim looking as uncomfortable as he always does whenever a camera is near. "Do I look that old? Do I look that skinny? Don't I look like a geek?" he always asks, peering glumly at Kodak versions of himself. "I don't like having my picture taken," he always states, with unnecessary vigour.

But there we were, Jim and all of us together in various permutations, assembled haphazardly into a collage at the foot of his bed, held together by that gift-wrap tape that releases easily, then affixed more aggressively to the smooth plastic with surgical tape cadged from the supply room by a nurse. Laura pointed, interested: "So that's Al, the brother, I think he's been here. And that's Mary. I recognize her. That's you, of course. Is that Shirley or Kathy? I can tell that's Jim, I think. I'm seeing a resemblance. So you were all together and everything was okay and then suddenly he got sick?"

"That's Shirley and that's Kathy over there," I said, "and we were all together and Jim was fine. These were taken on a Saturday. The following Thursday night he came down with the flu. The following Monday morning he was in an ambulance. The following Wednesday he was transferred here. He's been here nine days."

"That's scary." Yes, it is. Now you're getting it, I thought.

SIXTEEN

Al and Heidi, one of his four daughters, were leaving the hospital as I arrived next day, a brutally cold January afternoon. He threw his arms around me — Al, who once announced that he doesn't hug anyone but his wife and daughters — and I was so startled I hugged him back, forcefully. I'm fond of Al. Like his father who died in 1982, he has simple needs and finds full contentment in his family, doting on his wife and his daughters and their children. Like his father, he is fond of making occasional declarations that implicitly invite opposition and he made one now, loudly, in the middle of the street.

"We've just come from seeing Jim and he's getting better. In fact, he's watching TV right now." Heidi nodded and smiled supportively. I was shocked into silence.

Halfway across the road to the parking garage, Al stopped and turned. "By the way, I know exactly how our new kitchen is going to look. I got the idea from the waiting room. Can't wait to start renovating."

I couldn't wait to watch Jim watching TV. What a breakthrough this was. What a dramatic comeback. Enjoying TV, when only days before he couldn't seem to open his eyes for longer than a second or two. Maybe he had a goofy movie to distract and entertain him. I bustled up to the phone just outside ICU but was told it would be a few minutes before I could see him. "We'll call you." Hmmph. He was probably holding off for a commercial break, too enthralled by the TV show for company.

The waiting room was unusually vacant, only a pop can or two left behind like footprints, so I could have a good look around at the future of Al's kitchen. He is a very good carpenter, and he planned and built his home himself shortly after he and Shirley married. I studied the wall shelving and cabinets in the waiting room, free to roam, stepping back and shaking my head, unable to understand how any of it could have inspired him. In all the years of our friendship, I had never known that Jim's older brother favoured dark cabinetry with a high gloss and a touch of the rococo, that he imagined Shirley would enjoy preparing their meals in a room with the warmth and dash of an accountant's office. The whole thing sounded wacky. Still, Al would work it all out and I was certain the result would be fine. He tries to roll with everything life presents, and maybe he only wanted to take from the waiting room something that would propel his optimism about Jim forward. He would probably revise his kitchen plan before he got home anyway.

Al has always been generous with his carpentry skills. He helped us renovate our first house, through the worst of Jim's chemotherapy course, knowing his brother was very ill and trying to make things better with his hands, all he could do. One day, I was administering an enema to Jim while he lay on a couch in the living room, acting on advice from a doctor to help him deal with severe constipation, an unpleasant side-effect of all the toxic drugs. Al walked in from the bathroom where he had been installing a vanity and was faced by the sight of two men, one of whom was inserting a rubber tube into the rectum of the other. Al was unfazed. "Either of you guys know where I put my electric sander?" he asked.

The phone in the waiting room rang and because I was alone I knew it was for me. Permission to visit. I was ready to celebrate his improvement, sorry I couldn't bring flowers for the occasion.

Someone passing his cubicle might have assumed he was watching TV. A TV set that looked like a castaway from a cheap motel was parked beside his bed, the side away from the serious medical equipment. It sat perilously on one of those some-assembly-required rolling carts, the kind that quiver when touched. With much fussing over lines and tubes, they had turned him off his left side and onto his right, so that he could watch. I watched what he could have been watching. Had his eyes been open, had he returned just then to full alertness, he might have caught the climactic moment when the lion pounced victoriously on the gazelle, a foregone conclusion made even less engaging by a droning announcer who blathered on about the predator/prey relationship while images blinked across a screen rendered fuzzy and benign by the absence of cable. Jim's not a big TV fan anyway and always leaves the room when nature-by-Disney exposes its downside so I wasn't surprised that his eyes were closed. The death of Bambi's mother haunts him still.

A nurse explained the presence of the TV set crammed into Jim's cubicle. "We thought he might enjoy a bit of diversion," she said, "but he didn't seem to care one way or the other. He opened his eyes, several times, in fact, but he didn't demonstrate awareness. He didn't follow the images. When you and I watch TV, our eyes move. I think he was just reacting to stimulus." Then she fiddled with the antenna, trying to sharpen the image, perhaps assuming I would want to watch now. "Sorry about the bad reception. This is the only channel we can get."

Al had understandably supposed that because a TV was playing in the cubicle and that Jim was facing it that he must be watching it or could be watching it if he chose and he took comfort from this apparent evidence that Jim was recovering. I had an impulse to snicker condescendingly, then checked it, recalling vividly that I was the person who had been staring at the night sky days before when a voice from nowhere reassured me that "this is not his time." I had not shared that spooky revelation with anyone else, had not been as generous with the family in my desperate lunge at hope as Al had been. But I had been carried up to ICU by his elation, sharing his anticipation, and was now saddened and glum as I sat by Jim.

He remained moribund but perplexing, because he showed faint, almost immeasurable signs of revival, like opening his eyes at the TV set. His blood pressure was no longer alarming. He still required oxygen but somewhat less than before. Yet he showed no serious evidence he was on his way back, seemed to be hovering, remained in "critical but stable" condition because the system has no other language to describe human stasis.

I called Mary that night and asked her to break the sobering news to Al that Jim would not be lounging in front of a TV set any time soon, and I was grateful because I just didn't have the heart to disappoint him. But by the time they spoke, Al had already called Kathy who then called me, nearly tearful in her joy, and I was forced to bring her into step with reality. There was silence. "Well, maybe they'll try it again," she said. "Maybe next time he'll actually enjoy what's happening on the screen." Not if it's the same damn show with the lion killing the gazelle, I thought.

It was a while before Al got around to elaborating on the hospital-inspired vision for his new kitchen, and it had nothing to do with what I had seen. He and Heidi had found a magazine in the waiting room with some plans in it that called for simple, light-grained cabinets and counters. Heidi could help with the project, because she works for a company that makes kitchen cabinets and she could get a price break. Al could save even more money by installing them himself, with some help from the "boys," two of his daughters' husbands. The renovated kitchen would have no hint of the gloomy or the heavily-varnished baroque. No abandoned snack bags or water bottles littering the counters. No fake leather chairs with arms bleached by fretful perspiration. Shirley would approve.

SEVENTEEN

The first priority of any ICU is to prolong survival, in the hope that the patient will finally recover to the point where constant monitoring and supportive equipment can be withdrawn. Outcomes like these are considered wins by the ICU team, a dedicated but competitive bunch. Obviously, deaths are losses. But sometimes language clashes with healing. Sometimes staff will boot around common words but give them an echoing resonance that can hold unintentional menace. "Failure" is one of those words. I know what it means, especially here, and it is clearly never uplifting. It has unmistakable connotations. But coupled with "extubate" in the same sentence, and attached to the chart of a critically-ill patient in an ICU bed, it can be both confusing and unsettling. And potentially harmful.

It is a significant move to wean a patient from a respirator, to extract the tube, hence to extubate the patient. There is much discussion beforehand by doctors and nurses, and the decision is never taken casually. It is considered an important milestone in recovery, a step toward independence, and everyone raises a cheer at the prospect because it is grounded in optimism. This could be a win. Fingers are crossed.

But no one is happy when the breathing tube has to be reinserted into the patient's mouth. That is bad news.

Sixteen days after a paramedic placed the first oxygen mask on Jim's face in our living room, I was greeted by a nurse who announced that they had tried to remove him from the respirator earlier that morning. "But he failed," she announced, clearly disappointed. "He lasted for two hours off it but then he started having trouble breathing so we had to put him back on again." I had not been notified about any impending attempt so I was taken aback. She brooded like a parent whose child had blown the university admissions test.

A resident came strolling by and raised his eyebrows at the nurse, an unspoken question. "We extubated this morning," she said. "But he failed after two hours." The resident shook his head, sighed and moved on to the next cubicle.

All kinds of people seemed to know there had been an extubation failure that day because the phrase recurred for hours, bouncing through conversations like a basketball. No discreet whispers out of earshot. Why didn't they just use the PA system: "Hey, everybody? Listen up. We attempted an extubation. Jim failed. Repeat: We extubated, he failed." Jim had let the side down but they assumed he didn't know.

Wrong. He knew, he knew. He didn't know exactly what had transpired but he knew that he had failed something of consequence and there was a defeated sadness in his eyes when he opened them briefly to look at me. He returned my hand squeeze without energy, a gentle, resigned acknowledgement, then drifted away again. I was furious at the cloddish insensitivity of the staff and tried to reassure him that there would be another chance, that it wasn't over, that he had lost nothing.

The very nurses who had argued plausibly that the unconscious hear more than we think they do had now betrayed their
own wisdom. He may have failed the breathing test but they had
failed to imagine he could hear their vocal disappointment.

I have heard families rant about inconsequential oversights,
about the sloppy evidence that even professionals can forget the
small tasks that don't threaten life. I have seen families howl in
outrage at soiled sheets and empty water jugs and hair that wasn't
brushed, knowing that was where they could place their helpless
anger. It's never about the full bedpan. It's always about the pain
and the loss, and I knew that, knew I did not need any lessons in
pop psych to refresh my understanding of displacement. I couldn't
get pissed off at Jim's destructive illness, no point in that, so I
took my anger out on nurses who had behaved callously. They
were handy. They would do.

Tube out, tube in. The following day I stayed home to catch
up on laundry and phone calls and tidying, enjoying a shaky
illusion of normalcy. Mary and Marg, her daughter, Jim's niece,
offered to cover visiting and drove the hour from Oshawa. Late in
the afternoon, Mary called from the hospital with an update. She
was obviously fighting tears. "Sorry," she said. "I'm still upset."

She told me she and Marg had been at Jim's bedside while
several nurses were trying to force a feeding tube down his throat
with no success, he kept choking on it, and he was crying and
Mary and Marg were crying and everyone was upset and frustrated and the nurses kept trying to jam the damn tube in and
Mary finally stepped in to plead for them to stop and they did but
they told her the tube had to be inserted one way or the other, he
needed it, and maybe she and Marg should just withdraw to the
waiting room for a while, take a break, everything would be fine.

PATRICK CONLON

When they returned, the tube was in place, leaving them to wonder how much aggression had been needed to restore it, leaving
me to suspect the nurses were turning into bullies.

Next morning I arrived at the hospital feeling like Jack
Lemmon in *The Out of Towners*, ready to take names, list them,
driven by an enraged mission to find authority higher than theirs
and rout them all. Avenge their clumsiness and stupidity, one
by one.

I was sitting at Jim's bedside, wondering whether I could sneak
him out, when I heard "Good morning!" and looked up to see a
doctor approaching briskly: white coat, stethoscope, name tag —
the whole uniform. This one introduced himself as a thoracic surgeon and added a polysyllabic name which I promptly forgot and
then he said he was called in to assess Jim. He was a very large,
bearded presence who chuckled at the nurse and followed her
appreciatively with his eyes when she left and then approached
Jim with the gusto of a door-to-door window salesman. "How are
you, Mr. O'Neill?" he blared from the other side of the bed. Jim
had two tubes in his mouth and could not speak. He stared at
the doctor, and seemed to register his presence. I wasn't sure.
The doctor's question seemed pathetically rhetorical.

I drew myself up to my full height, still considerably lower
than his, and I bellowed at him across Jim, only three feet
between us, summoning all the collected and stored anger from
yesterday and all the days before it: "Take a look, doc-TOR! How
the hell do you think he is?" I'm sure they heard me in the lobby,
eighteen floors down.

He blinked, then smiled, confident, still ebullient. "Well, as
a matter of fact I already know how he is," he declared. "He's
better than he was when I saw him a couple of days ago. Look.

98

Look! See that? We've removed one of his chest drainage tubes, there were five, remember, and we've clamped another one." He was right. I hadn't noticed a tube was gone. I hadn't noticed one of the remaining ones was clamped. "We'll see how it goes. Maybe we can remove that one too. So far he's doing okay." With that, he gave Jim's immobilized arm an approving pat and left.

I sat there, long after he had disappeared like a dust storm. Jim appeared calmer today, opening his eyes occasionally. I sensed he was finally beginning to know when I was there, and I reflected on a campaign that had backfired. I had won and I had not won. I had recruited the nurses into our lives, secretly yearning they would do better if they knew us as people. He was no longer just another case. His ICU nursing team now knew him as Jim, called him Jim, but they took it personally when Jim couldn't tolerate the removal of the ventilator and the insertion of the feeding tube, wanted Jim to succeed, breathe on his own, not to struggle, hoped he could take a step closer to leaving, shared his disappointment, their disappointment, out loud. They had bet on him, emotionally as well as professionally. But I hadn't been fair, hadn't allowed for the possibility that by revealing us to them I had tacitly invited them to reveal themselves to us. He was Jim to them now. They knew many of the people in his personal orbit and they endeavoured along with him, endeavoured also for professional detachment always and sometimes failed, being first human and then practised. My anger was starting to wane. It's never about the bedpan.

EIGHTEEN

*T*wo days later, Jim suddenly started to bleed from his rectum, but no one on staff was alarmed. It's common for patients in an ICU to bleed occasionally. The body has endured a battering from the illness and then another battering from the rescue, with foreign objects inserted into various openings, some natural, some not. Oxygen is supplied by a machine. Nutrition is delivered in drips. Antibiotics upset the natural balance. The body finally rebels, often developing an ulcer or a gastrointestinal lesion.

He continued to bleed, on and off, for several days. The unit called in a GI, hospital shorthand for a gastrointestinal specialist, and he suggested a colonoscopy might be necessary to trace the source of the bleeding. In Jim's case, a stomach ulcer had already been ruled out, although no one ever explained why. It could be something else, then, even a polyp in the upper or lower bowel, and a colonoscopy was the only way to be certain. The GI was ready to go hunting on short notice. "We may need to investigate," said a nurse, using a phrase that resonated with unintentional threat. Later, I overheard her with a colleague: "We may have to scope him." .

There was a problem. Jim couldn't be called an ideal candidate for a colonoscopy, an invasive procedure that uses fibre optics to examine the large intestine. He offered none of the basic criteria, like a reasonable heart rate and stable vital signs, for an aggressive internal investigation. Even robust people quail at the prospect of having a tube with electronic eyesight shoved up the anus, the only logical point of entry until someone invents a kinder method. For many, the uncomfortable procedure is a good excuse to avoid doctors altogether. Ignorance trumps fear.

I gave standby consent to a colonoscopy, desperately hoping it wouldn't be necessary. It wasn't. The bleeding mysteriously stopped as suddenly as it had started. "Bleeding resolved" was the chart entry. I went home, relieved.

But then it started again the next day for no reason that anyone could confirm so the nurse called it "phenomenal." Now there were some frightening possibilities, including the presence of a cancerous tumour, that loomed in discussion with staff. Jim's father had died of bowel cancer. One of his sisters was being treated for colonic polyps that eventually proved benign but she had endured the initial what-if scare that accompanies every impending diagnosis. It might run in the family so everyone but Jim had endured a colonoscopy. So far.

That night, Norma was the nurse on him, small, cheery, smart, veteran Norma. It had been a day of fighting the worst fears, pushing them into a corner, winning all day until I was finally exhausted and sliding into panic. I began pacing in circles outside his cubicle, going around and around.

Norma watched me for a full minute. "You'll wear out the floor," she said. I could only stare at her, shaking my head. Then she stepped away from her desk at the foot of Jim's bed and stopped me. "What's wrong?" she asked.

It poured out of me then, all the grief and terror and frustration, some of it muted gibberish. I was fearful that he might have cancer again, trying to keep my voice down but railing at the latest setback, this bleeding that came and went, that had now conquered me because I knew it could kill him. "He could bleed to death. After all he's been through, he could bleed to death."

She touched my forearm and looked up directly into my face. "Don't trouble your heart, hon," she said. "They can fix that."

Then she stepped back and squinted over at him appraisingly. With the lights dimmed, he seemed to be shrinking subtly into the bed now, blending with the sheets, seeming as still as the wall behind him. "This one's going to make it," she said, and nodded as if to support her own claim.

"How can you know that?" I was snappy, all of my frustration in the challenge. "He's nowhere near making it. How the hell can you simply look at him and know that?" She gazed at him again. "I just know," she said, without turning away from him. No conceit or swagger in her voice. Only a confident prophecy from one ICU nurse who had lived through a thousand deaths and revivals. Gathered insight, one crisis at a time. "I always know," she added, "and I've never been wrong." With that, she quickly scanned the monitors beside him, nodded again, sat at the foot of his bed, and continued to watch over him.

NINETEEN

"*Mon pays ce n'est pas un pays, c'est l'hiver*." My country is not a country, it's winter. Gilles Vigneault's soaring anthem to a solitude framed only by snow and ice and wind is playing on the car radio, and I hum along with his gruff voice, bringing forward memories of my own Quebec childhood. I want to embrace and celebrate this place with no predictable geography as he did his, needing nothing but being with Jim. Instead, I scurry from warmth to warmth, to car, to hospital, to car again, to home and back, growing resentful of the dulling routine.

It is January 11, day 20 of the crisis, and he has not changed noticeably since admission, only rallying to consciousness in brief surges, gazing incuriously around, then drifting back to his own private burrow. In a small room with laundered air and a temperature that never varies from near-tropical perfect, where sweaters quickly become superfluous, he hibernates. I want him back, him as he was before, and wonder if we will ever again be who we were.

On this Saturday afternoon, stinging bright and cold, I have been halted at the phone outside the ICU because they're doing something in there, they don't say what — they never do, and they ask me to wait. But I have learned that they sometimes arrange patients for family visits, a practised ritual. Like attendants in a funeral parlour, the nurses bathe them and tidy them, expunge any nasty odours, so that they can be presented at their best, which is seldom very good but still on this side of death. I have decided I can't face the waiting room again, all those nervous faces and the etching boredom, so I retreat to the lobby to wait at a coffee shop next to a large window near the hospital's main entrance.

Outside the main entrance, groups of angry protesters are massing for a march on the American consulate down the street. They are here to denounce another looming assault on Iraq, their anti-America placards flashing a game of hide-and-seek around the very large white van at the hospital's main entrance. It squats defiantly in a rigorously enforced no-parking zone, and nothing identifies its purpose. I imagine that it is there to monitor the protest, its slab sides concealing equipment and perhaps even troops. Like unmarked police cars, it is probably one of those official vehicles that pretend to an innocuous presence, tricking no one with their calculated blandness. I turn from the counter with my coffee, hoping for a place to sit and watch.

All three poky tables have occupants. At one of them, a stocky man sits alone reading a paperback and he happens to look up while I'm scanning the tables for any sign of impending vacancy. He gestures to the chair opposite him and I sit, mutter thanks, and watch the protesters form a parade of sorts, shuffling reluctantly into position like school kids on a day trip. Two of them joust playfully with their placards.

We soon become winter companions, the stranger and I,

lost in our shapeless coats like old men while people hustle past us to and from the elevators. He says he is from the West, somewhere outside Saskatoon, and also a writer, he reveals with the tentative pride that marks unfinished work. He is writing a history of his family, early arrivals from Europe who worked hard, made a fortune from grain, lost it, remade it, lost it again, then opened a muffler shop that became a big chain that sprawled across the West, lost all that, up and down for generations, the bouncing from poor to rich to poor now ready to be chronicled.

We talk about writing, the drumming work of it, agreeing that the easiest to read is the hardest to write, followed by a comfortable silence and then ruminations about the weather and the anti-war march still forming outside. He reaches for his coffee and suddenly exposes a plastic hospital wrist bracelet. I can't help staring at it, suddenly aware he is a patient here. "Nine South," he explains tersely, and then elaborates. "They're doing some tests. I'm here for a few days. They want me to hang around until the results come back. But I'm not worried." Nine South, I wonder. I don't know the hospital that well. Cancer? Heart? Some gruesome and mysterious disease that Saskatoon shipped him east to confirm, a respectful nod from a small-town hospital to the resources of a wealthier big-town hospital? "I'm sorry," I say, resisting the urge to add a platitude about the gnawing wait for information.

He brushes my sympathy aside, a stoic prairie shrug. "See that truck out front?" He is facing me but his eyes flick to the fat white van, still blocking the view of the boulevard, the grand sweep of the wide street. "They can hear every word we're saying." He glances around the lobby. "Everything."

I wish him good luck when we part a few minutes later,

and glance back once before turning the corner to the elevators. He is absorbed in his book again. Up in ICU, cleared for entry, I ask Jim's nurse about Nine South. I'm curious: what do they do there? "Nine South? That's the psychiatric wing," she says, then smiles, teasing, and looks me up and down. "But don't worry. You're not ready for Nine South yet."

On this day of hard sunshine, echoing with its wails and discordant clanging, I am not certain she is right. I am only certain that war will happen. The white van tells me so.

TWENTY

*T*wo days later, a Monday, I was propped in the lobby again, this time shunning company.

Not surprisingly, the pace of a big city hospital quickens during the week, during the day, and it was obvious now. There was brisk purpose in the mood of the Mount Sinai lobby, propelled by visitors who bustled through because they had someone to see or something to sell. Two men in business suits greeted each other with practised weariness.

"How are you?"

"Busy. You?"

"Busy."

"Coffee?"

"Can't now. Got a ten, an eleven and a noon. Then down for meetings all afternoon. Six for drinks?"

"No good for me. Kids' soccer practice. Tomorrow?"

"I'll BlackBerry you."

"Done."

That ritual complete, they exchanged sighs and shook their heads with apparent regret, unable to conceal the self-congratulatory smugness beneath. It is now very important to be busy, and to be seen as being busy — the Victorian notion of justice come to 21st century commerce — and I'm surprised there isn't a Busiest Person of the Year award yet. I was busy waiting, watching the lobby traffic, content to idle until I could see Jim.

As kids, we counted barns to ease the boredom of long road trips. Here, I counted all the anxious faces, flashing by in flaps of wool and fur, and arrived at some distracting generalities.

Those who would spend their time at bedsides or for frightening tests had negotiated their presence in this building, wedged it into days with other, happier tensions, and they were pressed and uncomfortable. For them, this is an intimidating place. They did not want to be here but they knew they had to be and they were edgy. Some of them jabbed the elevator button several times, in the belief that aggression will summon cars more quickly.

Unlike most hospitals, Mount Sinai has never banned cellular phones except in a few places where they might interfere with sensitive medical equipment. But today their users seemed to be lurking furtively around lobby corners anyway, behaving as if they were performing illicit acts, sipping from cardboard coffee containers and muttering about appointments and health updates and visiting schedules. "I'm losing you. No, not her. She's fine, no change. It's you, I'm losing you. Wait. I'll call you back when I'm on the street."

The crowded elevator climbed slowly to ICU at the top, stopping at each floor as it often does on a busy weekday, and now I was jittery too, caught in the pace and mood of the lobby. I was weary of waiting. I wanted to see him.

ICU nurses don't need to hurry on any day of the week unless they're summoned to an emergency, which they had been down the hall from Jim this snowy morning. It was announced with the cheeriest of electronic melodies which meant it was very serious. I arrived at Jim's cubicle and then immediately stood aside as the crash cart went rolling by and when I was finally at his bedside I could hear but not see a cubicle curtain down the way close with a brief yelp from its rings as they skated along the metal rail. I heard low voices speaking urgently. Then there was silence.

Liz was the nurse with Jim that day and I asked her what she was doing as she fussed along the right perimeter of his body, the side with all the tubes coming from it. She told me she needed to free a kinked tube from beneath him, leading to a catheter, I think, and she was trying to lift him but an ungainly tangle of other tubes and lines made it awkward. I offered to help. She looked at me, obviously ambivalent, weighing her options. "It's okay. I can wait for one of the other nurses," she said.

Then she seemed to reconsider. She looked down at Jim, then at me, and nodded. "Let's see how it goes," she said. We carefully raised him toward his side, on an angle, me taking my cues from her.

He was tilted there, held against gravity. His eyes were closed and he seemed oblivious to the business around him. "Just hold him steady. Don't let him fall back. That's it. This will only take a second." She moved with easy efficiency, found the kink in the tube and straightened it. "That's done it," she said.

I had one hand on his hip and the other on his shoulder and I was gawking at the blue and white absorbent pad under his trunk while she straightened the tube that seemed to end at his groin. He'd had a bowel movement and I was searching his excrement for evidence of blood. The bleeding had spontaneously stopped the day after Norma's confident prophecy but I was still spooked. I was watching for signs of red and also for the black streaks that can announce a serious problem, and I leaned in.

As far as I could see, it was uniformly brown. His stool appeared to be normal, I thought, about as normal as it probably gets on an ICU diet, which comes from a bag hung on a trolley beside the bed and which is never tasty or fibre-rich. "Look at that," I said, pointing. Liz frowned. "We'll attend to that," she muttered. "I know he needs to be cleaned up."

Then, "Oh." She suddenly understood why I was staring, examined his stool and nodded in agreement. "Yup. Looks okay," she said. "Thanks for your help." We eased him back into place. He remained unaware, letting out only a small sigh when his head settled into the pillow.

I learned some things that day.

First: I learned how primed I had already become to be actively there for all of this, for Jim, not just a bystander through his ordeal but a participant in his care, there for the shit in the bed and the oozing from punctures in his body and the grotesque swelling, and there to place my hands on him in a way that was actually useful, even for a few seconds. Liz didn't ask for help. I was present, I offered, she accepted, and I was grateful. Finally, there was something I could do.

Second: I experienced something I had only read about, something that happens after the primal urge to ease the pain of someone close kicks in. I had watched parents tending their critically sick or injured children but had never really understood how they could be so apparently composed and methodical. Now I had felt it rise in me, that unspoken but clear invitation to something more than ineffectual hand-wringing. Once accepted, it results in an extraordinary but definite shift, a slight step back from the one who is loved but who is still no less loved for the step away. And I knew it resulted from some coalition of the spirit and the heart, and that it was a call to full presence. As I held Jim securely so Liz could deal with the tube, I realized that love can edit out all the smells and sights that normally repel, like a bowel movement in a bed, and then it goes to work. It is called professional detachment in those trained for it, who strive for it. In those deeply connected to the suffering person, those whom the system calls informal caregivers but sometimes dismisses as amateurs, it is unsentimental love that is channelled to action. All that matters is the doing.

It is judgemental and perhaps even trite to suggest that any life-threatening health crisis will always serve as a valid test of authentic love, separating those who would participate (that's love) from those who would withdraw (that's not). There is no test here. There is only the opening of a door to a place where anguish can actually intrude, where it can get in the way of the doing. At his bedside this day, I acknowledged it and embraced it — that confident sense of gentle but deliberate disengagement, that disregard for the messy and unpleasant by-products of his illness — in order to focus on the care, even a simple task, and I knew that I could do this and it became the unexpected sequel to that decision to ride with him in the ambulance on Christmas Day. All the way in, or not at all.

Third: I realized that Liz is like most nurses. They try to do everything, try to keep everyone happy, get annoyed with themselves when they fail, are hesitant when practical help is offered and are generally gracious about the accepting of it, when no disasters ensue. I knew I would continue to offer.

Fourth: I learned that life can come down to celebrating the colour brown, one bowel movement at a time.

ON MY WAY out for a coffee break, I passed an empty cubicle, its bed stripped and ready for the next occupant, and remembered the Code Blue call. Yes, it would have been this patient, I speculated, remembering only a man who seemed to be young, but I wasn't sure, someone on the periphery as I walked to Jim's cubicle, focused on my destination. The effort at resuscitation had probably failed and I thought kindly of him and of his family and of the people who had tried to save him, all of them gathered for the most human and most uncertain of missions.

TWENTY-ONE

*M*ore test results later that afternoon, from yet another resident, this one a woman who looked like Dr. Masur who had briefed me Christmas night after Jim had arrived. But, no, I thought — this isn't Dr. Masur. Is it? All the young residents were starting to look alike, talk alike. They all conveyed information in choppy, hurried sentences, probably animated by the release from text books and lectures and theories. They knew this is where the real work gets done, and they relished being here.

She rattled through a list of Jim's blood counts/blood pressure/ heart rate/respiratory responses and I nodded, already beginning to understand what they all meant. Then she turned to leave, paused and turned. "By the way," she said, "the HIV test was negative." She shrugged. "The result was slow coming back because of the holidays."

By the way. That's all it was to me, too. An afterthought. One more possibility crossed off the list. I felt no relief or satisfaction at a test result that was expected, unless it had now been determined after all these years that HIV can actually be contracted from a washroom door knob. I didn't feel superior or self-righteous either, in a relationship that has dared none of the so-called risky behaviours that ultimately killed dozens of our friends. We were too inhibited by childhood religious education and lingering Baltimore Catechism images of a milk bottle blackened to graphically represent soul-damning mortal sins like adulterous sex, too wrapped together to venture the complicating strategies of deceit, finally too tired for the libidinous stray, and we were monogamous because it felt deeply right and because the serious contemplation of anything else was daunting. Years of boogie nights spent snoring. This was just another test result. Nothing outrageous.

It was Dr. Bill McMullen that first day in Emergency who asked me if we'd ever had The Test, a phrase that still has a chilling resonance for gays because it can so swiftly boot logic aside. I told him that we had been monogamous since long before AIDS interrupted random passion, weren't needle users, never thought a test was necessary. We need to know, he had persisted, and he had gone on to explain that Jim's early condition was starting to mimic the kind of quick-moving pneumonia often found in AIDS patients with hammered immune systems.

Well, Jim certainly had looked the part when he was admitted to hospital, a poster boy for medical disaster that strange and mournful day.

I had given swift consent to the test, hungry for any answers the hunt might yield, and a sample of Jim's blood had gone off on Christmas Eve to a public health lab for analysis. I had forgotten about it until this casual aside from the resident at Mount Sinai weeks later.

By now, Jim's moments of wakefulness were extending, minute by minute, like the slow retreat of darkness on early spring afternoons. He seemed alert when I told him that they had done an HIV test and that the result was negative, no surprise. He stared at me, not reacting, and I was puzzled by his apparent indifference. Then I saw anger rising in his eyes, something so sharp and unexpected after all this time of feeble response that I gulped. "Sorry," I said, because I read him as we had learned to read each other over the years. And I knew what he was demanding to know, even if he could not voice it: "Would they have pushed for an HIV test if I wasn't gay?"

Not a question to which I had an easy answer. Nor was I completely reassured by official claims that hospitals now call for the test routinely, regardless of gender or sexual orientation, and that consent for it is sought from the patient when possible. But one ICU nurse told me there are signs in ordinary blood work results that can flag the possible presence of the virus. "We don't really need the test, except to be certain," he said, with a hint of smugness. "We don't really need consent." I didn't know whether he was bragging or just plain wrong. He was not calming.

Was Jim being touchy? Was I in those early days too eager for inclusion to challenge a hospital agenda that seemed sensibly grounded in a series of rule-out tests? Did I look back and feel I had reacted at times like one of those embedded reporters in the Iraqi war, trading an urge to challenge for a place near the centre of his care, surrendering effective advocacy for an illusion of control? Maybe, maybe, and yes.

TWENTY-TWO

"Better airway management." It sounded like one of those sober vows from the dais at an annual shareholders' meeting, designed to hint at bigger profits and to reassure investors that corporate diligence knows no limits.

"Huh?" was the smartest response I could think of.

It didn't faze Tom Stewart. He was moving hurriedly, as always, decked out in his hospital uniform of shirt and khakis, and he had stopped me in a hallway outside ICU. No doctor's white coat. That's for special occasions. It's Stewart's equivalent of formal wear.

He had come to a halt with a soft squeak from his rubber-soled shoes, a squeak that sounded like a small animal in distress. There was no preamble. "We want to perform a tracheotomy," he said. "We feel Jim will continue to need oxygen assistance for a while and a tracheotomy will result in better airway management."

"Huh?"

"It's a more efficient way of delivering oxygen. It also helps prevent long-term damage from being on a ventilator, from having a tube stuck down his throat all the time. It'll make him more comfortable. He's starting to be more alert so we'll ask for his consent before we do anything. See you later." Another squeak from his shoes and he was gone.

Two pieces of information, neither pleasant: it seemed Jim wouldn't be breathing on his own any time soon: and puncturing his windpipe would be the next phase in his recovery.

The days by then were spoons of tapioca pudding, soothing only in their predictability, all the little bites new routines dropping into play. Rising, feeding the dog, coffee, the call to the nursing station for any overnight updates, walking the dog, the drive to the hospital, the familiar bedside chair that always scraped the floor, the banter with the nurses, the anxious exchanges with visiting family, the drive home, feeding the dog, walking the dog, the canned ravioli (alternately, canned pea soup), the phone calls from friends and nothing to report except "stable" (alternately, "holding his own" and "hanging in"), the escape to TV — anything would do — the sleep, the rising and, now, the contemplation that he could possibly survive but that our immediate future would be counted in inhalations, one at a time. A hole in his throat would be the signal to settle in.

Mary was not surprised. When I called to alert her and the family to Tom Stewart's disquieting plan for a tracheotomy, she was sanguine. Except for rare moments, like the one after nurses tried to reinsert Jim's feeding tube, it was hard to read how she felt about anything. "I've been wondering when they would propose that," she said, drawing on her nursing experience. "It's just something they often do for patients who've been on a ventilator for a long time. It makes sense." Nothing made much sense then. I still had only the hope that improvements would be swift, that any day now I would arrive carrying a suitcase of his clothes to bring him home.

He had other ideas.

A couple of days later, Laura, his nurse for that shift, greeted me with some puzzling news. "It's very strange," she said. "He seemed fairly aware and responsive this morning so we called in the ENT guy, the surgeon who's going to perform the trach, to explain things and get his consent. But it was just like Jim suddenly slipped back. He seemed confused and disoriented. The surgeon got no response at all from him. He left without getting consent. We're not alarmed but we don't know what's going on with him."

Neither did I, even after a satisfying visit. He seemed fine, reacting to my words with careful nods and head shakes, apparently recognizing nurses with solicitous questions who drifted through, lightly squeezing my hand. I didn't raise the prospect of a tracheotomy or question his reaction to the surgeon's visit that morning. I figured his baffling earlier behaviour was just part of the winding track of his illness. He was coming and going from awareness now. Maybe the surgeon would return and find him in a lucid moment.

But late that night, the pre-war bombast on TV newscasts now silenced to moving lips by a remote-control button, I dozed over a mug of tea and thought about Jim and about the swerves of the day with him and about things not always being what they seem. Something nagged, something unseen and elusive hovered in the shadowy undercurrent of the day.

Then I remembered. Then I had it, an old image of grief and struggle and final acceptance. But I was still uncertain. I placed a whaddya-think? call to Mary who then called Al who then called Kathy who then called me and said, "You know, it makes sense ..."

The following morning, I was at the hospital early. Laura was with him again, entering notes into his chart. "I think I know what's going on," I said. She looked up, momentarily confused. "The tracheotomy. I think he understood the surgeon, I think he knew exactly what was going on, and I think he withdrew. He pretended he didn't understand." She nodded, and waited for more. "Just give me a few minutes with him," I said. She stepped back to the nursing station, watching him from a distance.

I pulled up the chair and sat and then hunched forward. His eyes were open. I took his hand and gave it a gentle squeeze. He squeezed back, tentatively at first, then with more certainty. This was encouraging.

I brought him up to date: Hope had eaten all her breakfast (always good news in a very old dog) but our walk had been short because of ice on the streets. Mary and John were coming in later, Al and Shirley would be in on the weekend, Firefighter Bob from across the way had cleaned a thick coat of ice off my car, Donna sent her love, promising to visit again soon. The stitchery of his life away from all of this.

Then: "Do you remember a doctor coming to see you yesterday, a surgeon who wanted to talk about doing a tracheotomy?"

Hesitation. Then a slow nod.

"They're proposing it because it'll help you breathe more easily. You know that, don't you?"

No reaction.

I took his hand, held it. "You're afraid of it, aren't you? You don't want them to do it."

Another slow nod.

"I think I understand why you don't want it. I think it's the right thing to do but it has to be your decision. No one wants to force you into this."

No reaction.

I looked away and then back. I wanted to be very careful about what I said next. "Is it possible a tracheotomy makes you think of Paul, the way you knew him in those final weeks before he died? Is it possible you think you're dying too?" Paul had been a much-loved older brother who had died of throat cancer more than twenty years before. They had given him a tracheotomy to help ease his struggle for air in his last days. It became a palliative emblem. The child of high promise, the hero to his youngest brother, the charm, the intelligence, the cars, the women, the marriage and the debris of its ragged end, the disappointments, the alcoholism, the worrisome disappearances, the grotty rooming houses, the contempt, the confusion, diminished in one final bed, tended by kind strangers who freed him for reconciliation while oxygen took an expedient shortcut to his lungs. I remembered, all these years later: Jim had watched him die, had seen his voice taken away, and he had never forgotten those final weeks at his brother's bedside.

He stared at the ceiling. I waited. Then, tears welled in his eyes. I could see the misery and the pain and the fear. A slow nod, a look away.

Fighting tears myself. "You're not going to die like Paul. That's not why they're doing this." A fierce whisper, desperate to comfort him, make him see that a tracheotomy could be a step closer to life, not death. It didn't always have to mean that death was next.

I let it go then, continued to hold his hand and talk about family, and left a while later to find Tom Stewart. "I need help with something," I said and then explained Jim's resistance.

Stewart responded swiftly. Within minutes, he showed up at

Jim's bedside and quietly assured him that he was doing fine, that the tracheotomy was only being proposed to help his lungs recover. I started to enlist all the nurses in the unit but word had already spread so they knew anyway and most of them in adjoining cubicles took turns, leaving their own patients briefly to boost the campaign, giving Jim reassuring smiles and encouragement. One doctor, a resident, stepped up to the foot of Jim's bed, raised a clipboard, waved it for emphasis: "Mr. O'Neill? Jim? You don't have to worry. In your case, a tracheotomy is not an end-stage procedure!" Jim looked bewildered.

"Not an end-stage procedure." The phrase started to float around Jim's cubicle like a tribal chant. But the team wasn't finished yet. It was time to close the deal. Betty Lynch-Powers was pressed into service.

She's the ICU chaplain at Mount Sinai, a gentle presence in the body of everyone's favourite aunt. She was seeing Jim for the first time but she'd been briefed and quickly went to work. While I stood on the other side of the bed, she sat as close to him as I had been a while before. He turned his head to her, he looked directly at her and she began speaking softly, holding his hand. "Do you know how proud of you your family is? Do you know what your grace and your courage have meant to them?"

I stepped back, entrusting him to her, feeling by now like an intruder, wanting to give them privacy, watching them engage. Hearing nothing, because by then she was silent and he was watching her, their faces inches apart, something happening between them that astonished with its power. She seemed to go to his silence and wait there for permission, then she was given entry by something in his eyes and what followed was as resonant and as clear as a dialogue, not voiced but seen and felt, their faces still and concentrated, his finally relaxing. It was a few seconds before I realized I was crying. She had reached him in the dark place where his terror lived, eased him away tenderly from its clutches. I had witnessed something extraordinary and moving, and I could only stand in awe. She kissed him on the forehead and withdrew slowly from his side. "He has a very strong spirit," she said. "Call me anytime if I can help." Then she left.

Next day, the surgeon appeared again. This time I was present. He looked too young to be allowed anywhere near sharp instruments. I waited across the bed from him while he efficiently explained the tracheotomy procedure to Jim, making the point that it would be quick and routine. "I've done lots," he said by way of flashing his credentials. Then he remembered the script: "In your case, I want you to know it's a therapeutic procedure. You're not dying." I made sure Jim understood everything the surgeon had said. He looked at him and nodded his consent.

The tracheotomy was in place within twenty-four hours. Jim appeared calmer. I should have felt comforted, gathered in the embrace of professionals who had answered the call for compassion and generosity.

After all, he was breathing more easily, the goal of the surgery achieved. He now had a round puncture in his throat, between his Adam's apple and his breastbone, and it was flanged with plastic with some kind of clip to secure the tube that led from it to a respirator. I could see a pale corona of dried blood that had seeped out from under the flange. Jim was receiving oxygen directly into his lungs, relieving any pressure on his mouth and throat.

He would still be in peril, of course. Hospitals cover themselves by reciting all the risks of any procedure, even the routine cuts, and I remained aware of them all along, even while I pressed the campaign to win his acquiescence and thanked the collective support that enfolded us.

He could bleed internally, acute infection could develop, his lungs could collapse, his voice box and esophagus could be damaged. In fact, he could take his last breath through that skinny tube stuck into his throat, an end-stage gasp. But the statistics claim that only five per cent of tracheotomy patients die. The odds seemed to be turning in his favour.

Still, doubt began to scratch at trust: had I complied with an agenda that could hurt him, even kill him? Did I say, go ahead and cut him because you guys know what you're doing, and I don't, not at all, but you're the only hope I've got so I'll play along because that's what I can do and because I need you to like me right now, need to feel I am a partner in this, need to feel I am one of you, need to feel not alone in this.

Of course. Those uncertainties were familiar terrain by now. I could bat them aside, subordinating them to the goal. But it was only when I looked at him, at his chest now lifting and relaxing without effort, at his face, at his eyes staring back at me, that I realized he could no longer speak, and I was chilled by my own blindness to one of the immediate consequences of any tracheotomy, by my failure to console him in his dread of becoming a mute.

I had somehow ignored that part, skipped past it to the goal everyone seemed to want, remembering Tom Stewart's argument for better airway management. It is so obvious a by-product of the procedure that it is not even mentioned in any of the literature on tracheotomies and their risks. It was never among my litany of dreads because this was all about us, them and me, looking after him and proceeding because the first imperative was efficient breathing.

But the same blade that had expedited the delivery of air to his lungs had also robbed him of speech. The hole was below his voice box. That was the outcome of the outcome, the unwritten coda to the surgery, and they could not know that they might have pushed him further from recovery by silencing him. How could they know that? I knew that because I knew him. Should the knowing of him and his needs have slowed me from so heartily supporting a tracheotomy? I wasn't sure. I only knew I felt like an accomplice.

TWENTY-THREE

L ate that night at home, I went rummaging for a particular photograph and found it tucked in a dresser drawer. It is black-and-white and tiny, probably one inch by two, and it sits in a flimsy cardboard frame edged in fancy scrollwork, with the sides folded back to keep it upright. It shows a very young boy, wearing glasses that are too big for his face but still failing to obscure eyes that are bright and engaged. The smile mixes joy and wonder and mischief. This is someone who has something pressing he wants to share because that has happened or this has been seen and it all needs telling, needs release, but he will wait, obediently, until he is dismissed by the photographer. On the opposite side, someone had written "Grade I" in careful black script now finally starting to fade. This is Jim at six. We were together for twenty years before he showed it to me. "That was the last time I ever smiled for a photograph," he said. I gazed at it that first night of his enforced silence and remembered something he had written soon after we met.

The early months of our relationship were marked by frequent arguments, all fuelled by insecurity, all ending in tearful reconciliation. We knew we wanted this messy union, knew it the first night we met. We just didn't know how to make it work and were often clumsy in the attempt. We had no role models then. There were no codes of behaviour for gays struggling to build committed relationships. The ones we knew, the relationships that had survived, were furtive and guilt-ridden, uncelebrated by family, condemned by churches, barely tolerated by a society that had decriminalized homosexuality only a few years before we met.

Late in our first year together, there was one prolonged fight that left emotional wounds too deep to fix with apologies and forgiveness. Things were shouted that could not be taken back. We said "goodbye" and believed it was final.

We weren't living together then but Jim had spent almost all his spare time in my apartment, the second floor of a duplex in central Toronto, so much time that I padded glumly around for days after his last exit, angry, missing him, grateful to have my privacy back. His toothbrush still sat in a glass in the bathroom. I resolved to toss it away every time I looked at it.

One morning about a week after he left, I was retrieving the newspaper from the front porch and my downstairs neighbour appeared at his own door, ready to leave for work. Tony was also gay and he lived quietly alone. He was an old man, easily forty-one or forty-two. We shared nothing but a building and the occasional hello. Tony had met Jim and he asked about him, about us, more out of courtesy than anything, and I was surprised at his obvious dismay when I told him the news because he usually seemed so reserved.

That evening, he called and explained that he'd done some counselling in the gay community and that if he could help us mend whatever had pushed us apart he would be glad to act as a kind of mediator. "If you want to try," he said, "I'll help you try."

I waited two more days and called Jim. He claimed indifference to the offer of mediation, hiding his discomfort behind bravado. But he decided to go along with the effort to prove our relationship really was over, that nothing could save it, that this ending was best.

That weekend, we met in the safe neutrality of Tony's living room, the match for mine above but furnished conservatively in tones of beige and grey. This was not promising. This was an old man hiding from his own homosexuality in a downtown place that mimicked suburban decorating values. What could he offer a pair of randy twenty-somethings trying to build on ground that was little more than libido and impulse?

All he did was encourage each of us to make a list of the things we were willing to undertake if we wanted to save the relationship, a list of good intentions that amounted to some combination of *entente cordiale* and leap of faith.

Jim and I met at a restaurant a few days later and swapped lists. The first item on mine was something pompous like, "I will try to work harder toward our mutual goals."

The first item on Jim's was, "I will try to be quiet in the morning."

It was then that I knew I didn't really want him to be quiet in the morning, muttered pleas to the contrary. I wanted him to be who he was. I wanted him to shake me out of my acquired pre-coffee grumpiness, to point with wonder at trees and shadows and birds as he did, to laugh at something goofy on the radio or in the newspaper, to share his unfashionable glee at just being alive, to talk about the small town where he was born and about what he cared about and how he could remember the names of all his many cousins and how the family's front door was seldom locked and how his mother taught him that you never turned away anyone in need and how there was always an extra chair at the kitchen table, just in case someone unexpectedly showed up at dinner time, and how the prospect of a serious relationship with another man terrorized yet thrilled him because it was so severely apart from the smooth and predictable patterns of his past, all that powerful adult generosity and kindness never extending without qualification to the forbidden or the different that he knew he was and that he wanted to accept.

He had come to believe that love is always conditional. He had concealed his true heart from everyone around him, from the benevolent aunts and the priests, from his parents and his friends, feared swift denunciation, learned to play alone and quietly, repressed the kid he had been at six, released it defiantly by scratching FUCK on the school washroom wall with the crucifix of his rosary at nine without being caught, and even now he ventured to present himself on a promissory note that began with a pledge of quiet in the morning. First, I will hide some of me from you, if that's what you want, if that's what it takes. I can do that, I'm good at that.

We continued to talk that night, on a bench in a nearby park, our lists discarded. Much later, near dawn, I said, "Aw, hell. Look what time it is. Good morning. Let's talk some more. You show me you, I'll show you me." The construction work of being us, not the him and the me separately anymore, was finally beginning.

But that was all fading, his voice sacrificed for easier breathing, his familiar and endearing conviviality another step away from returning, hushed by a tube that would remain in place forever or a week. Much depended. There was no list I could make that would change that.

TWENTY-FOUR

*H*is galaxy has cracked and banged and collapsed to this. There is no here here. There is only the steady puffing of the respirator and the murmuring voices and the strangers who slip in and out of his life like inquisitive phantoms, flicking on the headboard light, poking, assessing, flicking off the headboard light, moving on, and then the family, the brother, the sisters, their spouses, their children, all nodding and smiling reflexively, all eager to share any sign of improvement, even when there is none to see. He dozes under daytime ceiling fluorescents and then wakes suddenly in the later dimness to nightmares that chip at his pain, showing their assault only with his eyes and with slight frowns, dulled into submission by the drugs.

All this I can only imagine in the void between us, watching him watching me, him blinking slowly, a reflexive up and down of his eyelids, me alert and wary, the sum of us reduced to feeble hand squeezes.

The nurses see it too, the lethargy that seems to have layered his deep illness like congealed paint, and they are frustrated because there are no windows on this side of the Mount Sinai ICU and they tell me that light, real daylight, would help. It was only the luck of the draw that he was delivered to this cubicle on Christmas Day, a wall on one side of it and curtains on the other two.

They discuss. They want to give him back his day and his night, his light and his dark, each one distinct and following the other in expected order, to restore the essential circadian rhythm, the ancient tick of the internal body clock, understood even by prehistoric hunters before they left their caves in pursuit of meat. A room with a window would be a good idea, patchy views of the clear winter sky transporting him from this truncated reality.

I am certain he would soar to it because he loves his sunny days, the shadows of trees and flowers licking the warm garden earth in the backyard that he works with his hands, standing sweaty and victorious when a row of seedlings has tottered to life, and a window would be his gateway back to that and to us.

Norma nudges me to lobby for a move to a windowed room, citing current medical opinion that supports the value of daylight in recovery. "Give his world back to him," she says. Eva starts, "If I were you ..." Laura says, "It's a shame he can't enjoy the sunshine." She waves vaguely at the far wall of rooms, hints of the day outside sneaking past staff and visitors, teasing past the large nursing station. I see a squeezed piece of blue sky. I sense a reluctance in the nurses to advocate actively with the unit's bosses, as though unmarked lines of authority would be crossed. They all agree it would help if I made the request for relocation, stepping him into line for a vacancy on the window side of the unit. "Have a word with the charge nurse," Eva says. "Ask her to put his name on the list."

When can he be moved? I am advised by the charge nurse who has duly noted the request at the nursing station that it could take a week, maybe longer, maybe less. No one can say for sure.

She explains the variables: someone will die or someone will recover or someone will neither die nor recover but arrive in sudden need of close care, like Jim weeks before. "Some of our rooms have windows and some don't, so it all depends on what happens." Like everything else around here, I think, and then retreat, mumbling thanks, hoping that a room with a window will vacate for any of the possible reasons.

TWO DAYS LATER, I arrive in the morning to seek clearance by phone as usual outside the ICU, I am granted cheerful admission as usual, wash my hands as usual at the sink to one side of the door and go swinging around now-familiar corners — left, then left again past the nursing station — and briskly up to the threshold of his cubicle, by now an actor easing into a practised role, already shrugging off my coat, ready to smile at him, but stopping, puzzled and briefly disoriented, then withholding any cheer from the woman who lies huddled in Jim's bed and from her companion, a man who sits at her side reading a newspaper with those half-glasses over which people always seem to glare at the world with chronic displeasure, as he does now.

No one has told me that Jim has been moved. He is now across and down the hall, tucked around a corner in a room with walls and a door, a room normally assigned to patients who require isolation. Large windows span one wall, but I only know they are there because the daylight is struggling for entry behind tightly-closed blinds that stripe his bed. Salina, his nurse today, tells me that on this sunny morning, his first morning here, he has managed to communicate that he prefers the dimness. She admits she is worried about him. His vital signs are fine, she hastens to add, there is nothing medically alarming, but something is changing, she senses that, but what and why elude her.

He has positioned himself on his side, away from the daylight struggling for entry, not fetal but scrunched. He can't be comfortable lying that way but he has made a decision, I see that, I see a hint of his determination, and he gazes blankly up at me, his ground established, the heavy stillness of the room relieved only by a duet of the hospital ventilation system and his respirator and I touch his hand apprehensively, then encouragingly, but he ignores me. I wait, and watch. Who knows where the time goes? I fuss with the corner of a sheet so he cannot see my eyes fill. His limbs twitch, then relax, then, a few minutes later, twitch again. It finally becomes harshly clear and bright: he wants no here or there. He wants only an end to this. He is dying, and wanting to.

TWENTY-FIVE

*H*e was still withdrawn and uncommunicative when Mary and John visited him about noon the next day. I was at home. She left his room to call me.

"He's still twitching," she said. "I don't know why, but John and I have both seen it. And I'm not sure he's even aware we're here. I opened the blinds but it didn't make any difference."

"I haven't spoken to his nurse yet. What does she say?"

Mary paused. "Well, that's the thing. The spasms or whatever they are don't last more than a few seconds. They're over before I can get his nurse in for a look. She can't actually see him from where she's sitting. But she has to have noticed them, but she says he's fine, she's not concerned, she says no one's concerned. So I don't know what it all means. Maybe it's not serious. I think he could be having seizures but ..." Her voice trailed off.

Mary didn't know whether to go or stay, troubled by the gap between what she saw and what she was told, reluctant to abandon him in this uncertain state, but I assured her I was planning to be there later in the afternoon. He'd be covered. I would seek answers. She and John could go home, and they did, after staying until about 2:30. Mary called again when they were about to leave: "He's ... I don't know. I can't explain it."

The phone rang again around 3:30 and I lunged for it on the kitchen wall, eager to go, wanting to ignore it, but surrendering to its ring anyway because it could be important, and it was. It was his nurse, it was Salina again from the day before. "I was just heading in," I said. I had called her earlier. By then I was calling in every day. Told her then, as I always told all of them, when I'd be in.

"Don't come here," she said.

"Pardon?"

"Don't come here," she repeated. "He's being transferred back to Trillium."

"Trillium? When?"

"Right now."

"But what about the tremors, or whatever they are?" I was annoyed. "Has he been having seizures?"

She hesitated. "He's been assessed and he's stable enough for the transfer. He'll be leaving in a few minutes."

There had been no warning, not even a hint that he would be leaving Mount Sinai that day or even any time very soon. I felt that I was suddenly dropped into a hidden aspect of hospital life that is often discussed but never named, that shuts out all but a few, a mysterious province in which patient transfers are performed without apparent cause or purpose, mobilization plans drawn in accordance with rituals and practices known only to insiders. It was easy to suspect that the orders are executed by faceless strangers in some back room who jerk the levers of motion and change. He was leaving but no one at Mount Sinai had openly acknowledged that Jim might be enduring seizures and I could only trust that they knew what they were doing when the decision to transfer him had been taken. After all, they were my pals now. Weren't they? We had worked together through the treacherous loops of his crisis. Hadn't we?

Were they bored with him, the unpredictable theatre of his case losing its visceral kick? Had they suddenly stopped paying close attention to him, ignored any tremors and contractions, drifted to other patients with higher levels of dramatic urgency — or was it simply decreed that Trillium was now the best place for him, whatever his condition? Had it all come down to this bed here was needed and that one over there was vacant, a chancy game of checkers? If I had pressed them, and maybe I should have but an impulse to challenge was buried behind shock and fatigue, perhaps they would have said something like, "Yeah, we know about the seizures but our work is done. After all, he's breathing again, right? Trillium can take it from here. If he dies, he's on their watch, not ours any more."

And what would Mary think? Maybe she would assume I had been complicit in this startling decision to send him back to Trillium, easy to imagine after a tense exchange between us the week before. It had seemed after some casual chat with nurses that I might actually have some say in where he went next and I was hoping it would be Trillium.

"Why Trillium?" Mary had asked. "Isn't it better if he stays at Sinai? Wouldn't it be easier if he's in the same hospital, for follow-up and things like that?"

"Trillium is closer to where we live. It's closer to his friends," I said.

"But Trillium is a much longer drive for the rest of us, for Al and Kathy," she countered, her irritation obvious. It was true. They all live east of Toronto and Trillium is beyond the western edge of the city. Mount Sinai is downtown and would shorten their drives by at least half an hour. "Did you ever think about family, about what we might want?" she snapped. I'm his family too, I thought — probably even more than you are, whether you accept that or not. But I could not say it out loud to her.

"Well, this is just something a couple of nurses mentioned in passing. Nothing official. We may not have a choice anyway," I said by way of defusing the tension and restoring our uneasy truce. At that point, we were simply sharing information about him, wary with each other, holding emotions back. But she presumed I would be consulted before Jim was moved. So had I. As it turned out, we were both wrong.

Not feeling at all grateful, I thanked Salina for the information and for her care and for saving me a long round trip, muttered an acknowledgement when she wished us both well, and hung up, ready to drive west instead of east for the first time in twenty-seven days, ready to go back to where it had all started, to chase the ambulance carrying him again. I thought about calling someone at Trillium, anyone, with questions about the confusing news. That's when I heard an angry voice on the street outside the kitchen window, a shout only slightly muffled by two layers of glass, followed by another shout even louder than the first, evidence a quarrel was a starting to build.

Held from leaving by curiosity about the ruckus, I peered out at the sidewalk bordering the south side of our house, late enough by now in the sunny January afternoon that I could see all the stretching shadows of poles and trees grouped in stately progression on the empty street, all easing the transition to dusk. But one of the shadows was moving and it turned out to belong to a large person, heading steadily toward the setting sun straight ahead of him, and I relaxed.

It was just Henry, in loud and furious debate with himself as usual, this day heavily bulked with down and wool against the cold, a toque pulled low over his forehead to his bushy eyebrows and therefore looking even more fearsome than normal, his arms swinging calmly in rhythm at his sides as he lumbered without pause over the ice patches on the sidewalk. No one knows much about him except that he is apparently evacuated from his home every day by unnamed demons to plod the streets of our small neighbourhood, slapping his internal dissonance with strident argument as he passes the businessmen with their briefcases and the young mothers with their children and the old ladies with their winnings from the bingo hall who all know it is just Henry. He can show up at any time of the day or night but he means no harm and people sometimes say hello and when they do he always says hello back, in a quiet voice that borders on embarrassment, briefly on leave from his own war, politely waiting another half block along his chosen route before resuming verbal combat with himself. But all of us are always startled by his ferocious and steady engagement with the invisible enemies of his peace and there is unspoken agreement among his neighbours that this is who he will always be.

In that half-minute at the kitchen window as I watched him trudge west toward a sun that would soon disappear, when there seemed no order or even plausibility in what was happening to Jim, I thought I understood Henry better than any of my neighbours, knew that his impotent wrath mirrored my own just then, knew that if we just sat down together for a while he and I could easily find common foes and hurts and betrayals, joined by frustration and by a most certain flight of control from each of our lives. We could be partners in our campaign against heartless authority.

Do you know Tom Stewart, over there at Mount Sinai, I would ask? He used to be a friend. He's in charge. Let's go get him. Let's find him and yell at him.

No, let's not. Let's not engage in this enticing folly and turn anger into useless noise. Even in my churning distress, I had to accept that Tom Stewart and his colleagues had simply moved on and that therefore Jim had moved on and that now I could only try to catch up, like a commuter chasing a departing train. In gathering to help him anticipate and endure his tracheotomy, they had taken a brief holiday from their clinical facades and then stepped behind them again when their job was done.

I wished Henry well, wished an end to his own inner hostilities, but I knew his companionship would provide no comfort. I was on my own. That was the only position I understood right then.

I watched for him as I set out for the hospital, following his path by coincidence and not by plan, yet squinting from side to side against the glare of the sun ahead for another glimpse of him, even checking the side streets as I drove. But he had vanished, he was gone from the backcloth of my anguish, and I was thankful.

TWENTY-SIX

*T*iger Woods knows exactly how to hold a putter, and he has the tournament wins to prove it, but I don't and it doesn't matter anyway because I have no interest in the game except for a queasy fascination with a culture largely dominated by straight middle-aged white guys with the expansive bellies and confident chuckles of the historically sheltered. Woods may play better golf than most of the bumbling amateurs who strain to emulate his skill and panache but they still own the greens and the club houses, the essential parts, the pretty parts.

Still, it seems there are right ways and wrong ways to hold a putter and I was reading about one of the right ones now, imagining my thumb on the shaft and my feet in spiked shoes placed just like those in the magazine photo of Tiger Woods, boredom overtaking agitation as I languished in the cramped little room around the corner from the desk at Trillium's Intensive Care Unit. It was the same room where, nearly a month before, that first day, Dr. Neil Antman had announced to Donna and to me that Jim was likely to die.

Today I had finally turned from studying the scenic print on a Kleenex box to a tattered golf magazine. I had already finished the Reader's Digest with its stubborn fondness for kids who say awfully cute things and with the cover sticker that says Do Not Remove. A wrinkled newspaper to its side engaged me long enough to confirm that today was January 21 but I had discarded it, in no mood for the pious front-page swagger of a U.S. president who wanted to take his country to war, claiming a just and rational campaign for global consensus but deceiving no one with his real intent — to inflict punishment on the heretics who had presumed to topple two cherished temples of his people's wealth. With life outside this room steadily reducing to soothing absolutes, apparent among them the wrong way to hold a putter and the right reason to go to war, I could only embrace the maybes and all the other twists and sways of ambiguous reality, sinking at the moment into a couch, so weary and debilitated that my chin was level with my knees.

I had been waiting nearly three hours to greet Jim's arrival from Mount Sinai. I had again driven the long, wide stretch to Trillium, past the Hydro corridor disguised as a fanciful meridian and past the old farm orchards now banked high with snow, a month deeper in winter but not yet hiding the suburban bungalows behind them. I had risked a speeding ticket on the worried assumption that the ambulance carrying him might get there before me and that my absence would add to his displaced bewilderment. I had sprinted and huffed up to the desk in ICU, wheezing my inquiry, asking where his room was so I could see him right away but they could only tell me that he was still in transit and they had cited rush hour as a possible explanation for the delay and why didn't I just take a seat in the waiting room and wait for their summoning phone call. He should have been here by now, I had fretted. Maybe something happened. Could they call someone?

Dr. Anant Murthy had come around the corner at that point, blinking at me in mild surprise, then swiftly recovering and confirming that, yes, Jim was on his way from Mount Sinai, with a hint of wonder in his voice that Jim was still alive after the dicey transfer from Trillium that he had recommended on Christmas Day. "You can help us settle him in when he arrives," Murthy had said, in a bid to ease my apprehension but not succeeding, only masking it temporarily, a lozenge dulling the sharpness of my anxiety.

I had headed for the large family waiting room downstairs from ICU with some hope that it might have changed from the unwelcoming afterthought it had seemed all those weeks before. But it was still gloomy and unreceptive. From an empty side room there, normally reserved for family consultations, I had called Mary and given her the news of his move, asking her to pass it along to everyone else, ranting about the depressing familiarity of the hospital, all the shadows and dark corridors a bleak reprise of that first night and its dreadful foreboding. I had yelled at her that it was all the fucking same all over again — knowing that "fucking" had never been in her vocabulary but not caring. I had gone on to rant that nothing had changed, that all the same play-ers were still in their places, that the woman at the snack counter still smiled at everyone who passed, that even the cleaner who had predicted snow for Christmas that first night still hummed as he tidied the lobby, that Anant Murthy was still mantled in good cheer and that he had suggested I might be useful but that all I could do was wait for Jim to arrive, never a prized skill of mine and especially not now when Jim was between there and here.

"Trillium," Mary had said, flatly. Then I heard a rustle and her voice again, muffled: "John? Jim is on his way to Trillium. It's Patrick. I think he's upset."

After the call, I had roamed the halls to kill time, too agitated to sit, hating all of this and all of them, showing up at the ICU nursing desk from time to time, testing their tolerance with questions to which they had no answers, until, finally, Anant Murthy had suggested I could wait in the small room where Neil Antman had once told me Jim was dying and where Tiger Woods had improved my stance in a game I would never play.

"His vital signs have been stable and except for the seizures it was an uneventful transfer. Here's his chart." I tossed the golf magazine aside and heaved myself off the couch and around the corner, coming face to face with two uniformed paramedics in conversation with the charge nurse, Jim lying motionless and small on a gurney to one side, the formal ritual of the handover wrapping up.

"How is he? Did the trip go okay? I'm his partner. He's been very sick, you know. It seemed to take you guys a long time. Did anything happen?" All of this released like compressed air.

One of the paramedics stepped forward. I recognized the voice I had heard moments before, the voice dispassionately reporting Jim's condition and his seizures to staff, but it changed for me, became suddenly sympathetic and reassuring. It belonged to a burly man who said, "Don't worry, he's doing fine, the trip went well. They'll look after him." He turned to assist the final move of their patient, from the gurney to a bed, then turned back and smiled. "Good luck to both of you."

I hovered, nabbing Anant Murthy on his way to Jim's room opposite the nursing station. "I'll help you settle him in like you suggested," I said, eager to be part of his care again. "I know about the seizures in the ambulance." Murthy looked at me and shook his head. "We're too busy. Take a seat around the corner again.

He's still having seizures and we don't know why. First thing we have to do is try to get them under control, and you can see him when we've had a good chance to assess him." All of which left me questioning why no one at Mount Sinai ICU seemed to have notified Trillium ICU beforehand that the patient heading their way was demonstrating spasmodic and involuntary movements. Or maybe they had. I didn't know. I withdrew to the claustrophobic room again to fulminate over the acceptable limits of clinical stability when transporting a patient from one hospital to another and stared at my knees and a forgettable watercolour on the wall until Murthy summoned me about an hour later.

He and I sat in a short corridor behind the nursing station, he on the edge of a counter and I on a hard chair, glad for relief from sagging springs, an X-ray on the big light box beside us, and I was squinting at it, sorting the light from the dark parts, and wondering why I was being shown a picture of Jim's lungs. Murthy caught my reaction and said, "Relax, that's not Mr. O'Neill. That's another patient." I could only conclude from the way he said "relax" that he assumed I knew the X-ray revealed bad news about a patient who was not Jim. I was uncharitable in my private relief.

Murthy then went on to describe Jim's condition as serious, universally assumed to be a shade better than critical, and told me that a neurologist was on his way to help figure out the cause of the seizures but that they were administering Dilantin, an antiepileptic drug, to control them for now and that I could see Jim, but only for a minute, which I did, hovering over him solicitously, forming a silent prayer while he slept.

Then I left for home to brood with Hope, our old dog, while trying to be grateful for his survival so far, despite the mysterious seizures, the tracheotomy, the heart attack, the possible stroke, the lungs still barely working and only with constant support, the demolition of his now brittle and scraggy body, the retreat of his spirit into silent dejection, and I didn't try to halt the descent of my own indignation into melancholic self-pity.

TWENTY-SEVEN

*J*im had no further seizures overnight, and two bedsores.
That was the important news when I arrived to visit him
early the following morning, having spent hours contemplating the old plaster pattern on the bedroom ceiling, the loops and
cursives revealing a heavy hand but a whimsical soul. We had talked
about replacing it with the conventional smoothness of drywall but
had never summoned the heart to erase someone's playful legacy.

The cause of his seizures remained a puzzle but staff had
decided to defer investigation as long as the Dilantin they were
administering kept any tremors under control. They had other
priorities. The bedsores, for instance. The bedsores demanded
immediate prosecution and judgement.

The nurse assigned to him wasted no time getting to her
point. "He had a fairly quiet night. Did you know that he has two
bedsores? He came back from Mount Sinai with two bedsores."

A nearby nurse overheard her colleague. She was keen to cor-
roborate. "I remember him," she said, with the careful resolve of a
trained witness pointing at the accused in a trial. "He didn't have
any bedsores before he went to Mount Sinai. He didn't develop
them here."

All said just in case I was wondering about the bedsores, which I wasn't and hadn't even considered in the mix of woes he was already enduring, only vaguely aware of irritation to parts of his skin that seemed to be caused by the tape required to hold various tubes in place. Bedsores had somehow never made it to my list of worries. A third nurse shook her head in dismay. "One of them is really serious," she said, "the one on his lower back."

It was clear no one at Trillium wanted to pardon the bedsores. Jim was welcome. The bedsores weren't.

Nor are they welcome anywhere, of course — and for good reason. They're ugly, they're painful and they lack the implicit nobility of wounds inflicted by accident or violence. They do not invite heroic rescue or flashy intervention, and few doctors would add "treating bedsores" to their accomplishments. They are usually condemned as humiliating lapses in care and they are the iconic wounds that send news crews into nursing homes to probe alleged abuses. They summon images of helpless octogenarians languishing in their own urine, the victims of cruel neglect, or of Third World children bypassed and forgotten by modern medicine, their suppurating ulcers provoking outraged response. They are considered preventable. They are very slow to heal and require frequent inspection, cleaning and dressing changes. They are the pesky ghosts of Western medicine past, come to rattle their chains at a dazzling 21st century system that wants to boast about its successes and disown its embarrassments. With biblical flourish, each one by its mutilating presence mocks the folly of pride.

A bedsore develops when blood supply to the skin is cut off by constant pressure in a bed or a wheelchair and it can develop in two or three hours, depending on the condition of the patient.

As the skin dies from lack of blood, the bedsore starts as an irritated section of skin that eventually turns purple and then opens as it breaks down, inviting infection that can quickly travel to muscle and bone. That's when things can get nasty and complicated. That's when death can result.

But there was something else underlying the swift and vigorous denunciation of Jim's bedsores by the Trillium ICU nurses, something that lingered in the air, and no one voiced it but I knew what it was. He had been transferred from the great downtown Mount Sinai back to a suburban hospital, from the so-called A team back to the B team, the B team trapped in glib public assumptions about varying levels of care. He was maimed by skin ulcers that they believed shouldn't have occurred, wouldn't have occurred on their watch. There was strutting satisfaction on their faces, in their certainty, in their competitive disdain. They made no effort to hide it.

I could neither argue nor agree with them. They made it impossible to engage directly with their unspoken judgements. Besides, they could also be both right and wrong about Mount Sinai's culpability. Right in their conclusion that Jim's bedsores had originated there. Wrong in their verdict that the bedsores were confirmation of oversight or incompetence.

My anger at Mount Sinai had carried into his first day back at Trillium, anger at the cavalier way they had apparently flipped him back like an illegal refugee. So I could easily have joined any of the nurses' tacit bragging, and built a new Trillium alliance as a bonus. But I also remembered Jim had required complete immobilization that Christmas Day at Mount Sinai in order to save his life, hooked to a last-ditch machine that promised nothing but an attempt. Like all of his other organs, his skin was in failure and he had remained paralyzed for days. He had been a textbook candidate for bedsores. I wanted to see them.

I waited until the following day, when the nurses were a little more relaxed and chatty, when it turned out that Linda was the Ken Follett fan and Jodie was the depression glass collector as well as one of the unit's unofficial experts on wound care. She was Jim's nurse that day and she had to excuse herself in the middle of our chat about the colour variances in old glass because his daily dressing change was due and I told her I had never looked at Jim's bedsores, hadn't even known where and what they were, and wanted to. She blinked, clearly a little thrown by the request, puzzled that anyone outside the profession might actually want to witness the cleansing and treatment of smelly lesions, a ritual not likely to feature in anyone's favourite TV medical drama any time soon. But she consented, no doubt indulging eccentricity in the interests of maintaining peace, and she tactfully withheld any concern that my stomach might not be up to the view.

We stood over him, the sun bouncing into his room off the snow on the lower section of roof outside his window, his eyes moving between each of us. I gently squeezed his hand. "Okay if I have a look?" He raised his eyebrows. "At the bedsores." It was clear he didn't know what I was talking about. I waited until he nodded, still obviously confused by what there might be to see. He didn't know he had bedsores. He only knew he ached. He nodded because he trusted me.

The bedsore on his elbow capped the joint like a scarlet yarmulke, as though he'd accidentally brushed a hot stove burner with it. Jodie was quick and efficient, cleaning it and then replacing one dressing with another. With help from another nurse, she then raised him to his side and over on a slight angle to change the dressing on his tailbone wound, the more complicated of the two. Its dressing was broader than the open spread of a very large hand. It seemed heavily padded with gauze. She gently peeled the layers back, small portions at a time, trying to spare him sting, revealing first a wide radius of red, smooth skin, then skin that was purplish, slightly mottled and uneven as more was uncovered, then a ragged outline of black tissue, and finally she exposed the raw centre of the wound, a gaping crater the diameter of a hockey puck that seemed to extend deep into his body in swirls of pink and red. I could see a small patch of white bone at its base, and he moved suddenly, involuntarily, as I looked and then leaned in, and I was caught briefly by an optical illusion because the bone itself seemed to shift under the sinew, rather than the sinew shifting over the bone, and it was radiantly white, so white that I marvelled at how white human bone actually is when it is still enclosed by a living person, not the chalky white of skeletons but glistening with a sheen that seems to emit its own light. He made no sound as Jodie proceeded methodically, his discomfort blunted by drugs. She began with a careful inspection and cleaning.

She paused and pointed. "See that? That black area is necrotic tissue, dead tissue. That's a potential source of infection," she said. "I'll have to deal with it, snip it away with special scissors. That's called debridement. I'll attend to it later."

I was relieved that I did not recoil or even flinch and I wanted to prove to her that I was okay with all of this, at ease with witnessing the harsh and repugnant evidence before us, the by-products of his ruin, ready for the casual chat of two people focused on a clinical task, privately elated by enjoying that sense of slight detachment again, loving him not less but better because of this useful distance in his care.

"Ever heard of medical maggots?" I asked.

It was out before I could stop it and there was nothing to do but respond to her raised eyebrows. I told her I had read somewhere that so-called medical maggots are enjoying a comeback, and did she know that they are sometimes deployed by American hospitals to cleanse stubborn wounds like this, using the most basic of natural skills to consume dead tissue, not a pleasant notion and perhaps inappropriate if not absurd to raise just now, but still a nice change of image for the slimy critters, I thought, as they go about their assignment of proving that technology and chemicals don't have to be the only healing tools in the kit. "Gross," said Jodie in mock disgust, and finished covering the wound with a fresh dressing.

At first, it was bravado and curiosity that impelled me to look, a need to prove I could, to myself and to them, and a need to understand the cause of the nurses' clucking. But I also knew as I gazed into the deep gash at his tailbone, almost symmetrical in its violation, that I had a yearning to link with him as closely as possible, with the core of his suffering, to meet and touch and understand all that had gathered to hurt and defile him, the visible injuries as well as the concealed, another assertion of my early choice to be there for all of it and to do what I could, to be an informed partner in his care and to go to him if he could not come back to me yet. I knew again that I would be there even if my final memory of him was that glimpse of shimmering bone or there if I could see each bedsore close and heal a centimetre at a time, to mourn or to celebrate, but always present for the proceeding awfulness of this event, its ending still uncalled.

At that moment, it did not matter that he had bedsores. They were being tended. It did not matter who or what had caused them. That was no longer important. It only mattered then that he was still alive. For now, nothing that wriggled and crawled would have him.

TWENTY-EIGHT

ost pens used in hospitals are cheap drug company hand-outs and pen collectors like me have no interest in them except perhaps for the ones stamped "Viagra" because they're still good for a snicker but I was now holding a vintage Parker 51 fountain pen and trying to explain its allure to a perplexed audience of one at the weekly St. Lawrence Antique Market the following Sunday morning.

The Parker 51 was announced in 1939 to mark the 51st anniversary of The Parker Pen Company. Or it was named by company president Kenneth Parker to commemorate a dinner he once enjoyed at Toots Shor's restaurant, whose famous New York address was 51 West 51st Street. Or it was inspired by U.S. Highway 51 which abutted Parker's Wisconsin factory. Collectors have been known to quarrel over which version of corporate lore is closest to the truth. The pen wasn't in full production until 1941 because the company wanted to thoroughly test it in various markets first. Over the next three decades, it became the most popular fountain pen in history and rumours say more than twenty million were sold, many of them passed down from father to son like family keepsakes. It was officially retired by Parker in the early seventies but remains a venerable classic, sought by enthusiasts who spend hours vigorously defending its merits on internet pen discussion boards.

Hans is not among its fans and, in fact, finds the Parker 51 a rather plain pen whose charms elude him but he is curious about a lot of things so he gamely mustered enthusiasm about this particular 51 that morning, an example in black with a gold filled cap, all the while discreetly concealing regret over his decision to ask about it in the first place and wondering why the hell Carole hasn't arrived to rescue him. He and Carole are old friends of ours. They've been trolling the market every Sunday for almost as long as Jim and I have, and Hans has a passing interest in fountain pens. He tends to favour those that aren't bashful but assert themselves with fat nibs and flashes of gold.

It is fair to call the Parker 51 an unadorned writing instrument that makes no claim to elegance. With its sleek and functional simplicity, it is a sturdy example of old-fashioned Yankee restraint. Even its nib emerges shyly from under a V-shaped hood, revealing only the tip but hiding nearly half an inch of solid gold. Although it was available in fancier versions, most buyers chose a Parker 51 that came with a gold-filled or chrome cap that clipped prudently to a shirt or jacket pocket, seated firmly on a plastic barrel that was usually a modest black, grey or burgundy, the favoured colours for a sober business class. Users of the first-generation Parker 51 had to remove a small cap at the end of the barrel and then draw ink from a bottle by activating a small piston. It was replaced in 1948 by a model in which the whole barrel unscrewed to expose a pliable storage sac caged in metal which was squeezed three or four times while dipping the nib in the ink, a trusty filling method that remained in place for the rest of the model's life.

Dear God. Will he ever shut up?

Just when I was about to slide smoothly into an illuminating sidebar about available nib sizes and the value of Parker date codes and my hunt for a rare see-through demonstrator, just when I noticed that Hans eyes were starting to glaze and his attentive nods were becoming robotic, I turned to Richie and asked him whether $50 was the best he could do on the pen, given its scratches and the dent in the cap and all, and whether his bid for the apartment had been successful, the one he had talked about the week before, the one with a spare room for storage, and yes and no were his answers.

Richie is one of about eighty dealers who set up their tables every Sunday morning before dawn and who spend the rest of the long day trying to persuade browsers that all this used stuff, much of it made last year but some of it made more than a century ago, is worth a second glance. Prices are always flexible in this graceless sixties box with the echoing hardness of a high-school gym, which squats across from the old farmer's market that once housed Toronto's first brick town hall and just south of the gracious building with the grand ballroom where Jenny Lind once warbled to an audience of rapt Victorians.

The antique market and its population have been part of our personal community for more than ten years, a forty-minute drive from our small neighbourhood but no less resonant and endearing, and the dealers share their lives with us, their lives of broken trucks, broken hearts, lost deals, found treasures, hit-and-run thieves, boorish customers, fights with their kids or boyfriends and the discouraging gaps between shoppers during which they stroll and assess each other's wares and carp about the weather. They all seem to live on the edge of financial chaos, the dream of a big score the only bait that keeps them in the game. They are more than peddlers. They look after each other, consigning merchandise to those of their colleagues who some-times can't assemble the money to stock their tables and sending customers to Mike or Danny or Stanya or Blake who might have something they don't have and who could be having a bad day. When Willem died after years as a dealer, they got a photo of him and built a modest shrine to his memory that sat in place on his regular market table for weeks while his son sold off what remained of his stock and spoke fondly of his father to anyone who asked about the man in the picture.

Many of the dealers asked about Jim this morning, knowing he was ill, knowing we're always there together, every Sunday without fail, buying this or that, always imbuing the transaction with more than an exchange of cash for things because we like most of these people. They are outsiders with none of the usual buffers and nets, eccentrics and misfits scrabbling to meet car payments and rents and food bills by buying and then selling the flotsam that bobs in the wake of death or boredom or despera-tion. But they sensed that I was lonely without Jim, felt mis-placed in this familiar building where he was almost always in sight, where if I lost him Ed would stand on a chair next to his table and shade his eyes like a sea captain searching for land, then point and holler at Jim if he was successful.

This raucous bazaar had become my only escape, all my days spent with him at the hospital and my evenings at home on the phone with family, calling Mary first and asking her to pass updates along and then my own sister in Ottawa who always offered to come and stay with me but I discouraged her because I only wanted Hope for company, and then Bron and Murray, our elderly friends who live on a hill in the country and who feared the winter roads so they didn't visit but waited for news to help quell their overwhelming anxiety. I blathered on to Hans about the Parker 51 because the pen and the market had nothing to do with bedsores or heart rates or tracheotomies or feeding tubes. For two hours a week, it was almost possible to ignore the tumorous dread that had settled companionably in the pit of my stomach.

Darlene was seated behind her table in an old fur coat, her customary defence against the winter drafts. This day I bought a magazine rack from her. It was a wacky gizmo that looked like a fugitive from a French bordello and it perched precariously on tiny curved brass legs, with a handle that allowed transport from room to room and some kind of clamp with a pull-cord that kept periodicals from spilling out while it was carried. The word "Journals" was overlaid at a rakish angle in elaborate brass script on its faded rattan side, just in case there was any doubt as to its purpose. I chose it for a friend with an affection for the quirky but Darlene drew a line through the cardboard price ticket and wrote a cheery note to Jim on the other side. Next, there were five glass plates I thought Jim would like, green and nicely ground, bought from Israel whose entertaining geisha-style eye makeup was set carefully in place as usual but whose hair this time was an arresting shade of carrot red that challenged the gold brocade of his vest. He asked $15, I offered $10, he accepted $12 with good humour, as usual. Like Darlene, he asked about Jim, asked how he was doing. "Holding his own," I said to both, with no idea what that colloquialism meant or even its derivation but knowing that it conveyed the universally understood message that nothing had changed.

The same solicitude was offered on my daily walks down the street with Hope, slow ambles in deference to her old age and the perilous ice on the pavement. I was never far from tears then but pressed them down and moved on, passing neighbours who would ask "How's he doing?" and then nod when I advised that he was holding his own, the words by now flowing into a practised chant, the only answer I could find for kind people eager to know of any variation for the better or the worse, people who had nothing in common with the dealers at the market downtown except our presence in their lives and the terrifying certainty that every life is held from sudden illness by the flimsiest of strings. What happened to Jim could happen to them, to any of us, they knew that, feared that, and his swift and dreadful plunge reminded them of their own frailty, the older ones especially, and some of them needed him to recover, would use any good news about him to inflate their own day with brightness, something he would be happy to know even as he winced at the notion of being anyone's amulet.

That Sunday morning on his way to Mass, Ken pledged another prayer for Jim to Saint Theresa who had not failed him yet and Janet said she would make some of her famous scones when he came home and Barb next door and Candace down the street both promised dinner — "You have to eat!" — always delivered to the door on china plates that were stacked in clean piles for later return. But there was no need to return the large tinfoil pan to Brenda, she said, when she showed up one night with 15 fried chicken legs, giving the pan a dangerous sag in the middle with their weight, and she apologized, slightly embarrassed, saying that it was probably too much but at times like this it's what she does, it's what she can do, it's all any of them can do.

Some friends maintained a worried vigil and were always edgy and even disappointed when they asked about him in frequent phone calls because "holding his own" did not satisfy their expectations. They wanted the quick and soothing fixes of their only experience with serious crisis, TV medical dramas that deliver resolution in 60 minutes less commercials, and they were mystified when there seemed to be no change from day to day. Why isn't he better yet? Why isn't he home by now? What's taking so damn long? Where's the fast-forward button?

I had stopped Neil Antman in a stairwell a week after Jim's transfer back to Trillium, knowing by now that doctors always had to be ambushed for answers. Their chronic state of haste kept them running, and I was never certain to or from what but always suspected it allowed them to skip past any threat of emotional messiness. I needed a doctor's opinion of Jim's status, needed to know the full reality of "holding his own." Antman sighed and leaned against the wall, glancing at his watch. "Get ready," he said. "His odds of survival are improving but he's going to be here for a very long time. If he makes it." Then he heard his name paged — "Sorry" — and he was gone.

I headed directly for the hospital from the market that Sunday — after a quick lunch with Hans and Carole at a nearby Tim Hortons during which further discussion of the Parker 51 was excluded, no doubt to Hans' relief — taking the expressway west, the same expressway used by the ambulance that had travelled east, the other way, for the Christmas Day transfer to Sinai weeks before. I left the green glass plates in the car when I parked but I was impatient to tell him what I had found, impatient to share all the names of dealers and neighbours and friends who had asked about him since yesterday. I pulled a chair up close to him and began to talk in a calm voice but eager to help him refasten himself to his life away from here.

I rambled on about Hope's understandable but frustrating aversion to bad weather and the friendly jousting with Israel over the price of the green plates and the note from Darlene on the back of a price ticket removed from the goofy magazine rack I bought for Roger and the Parker 51 I didn't buy from Richie which was just as well because I already own more than forty of them and Ken's allegiance to Saint Theresa who always comes through and my lunch of a bran muffin and coffee with Hans and Carole.

Speaking of food, I said, Janet from down the street promises to have some of her terrific scones ready whenever you want and you remember Norma, she's that nurse from Mount Sinai who urged me not to trouble my heart, I think I told you about her, Norma called me last night to find out how you were doing. Wasn't that thoughtful?

I was suddenly aware when I waited for reaction that he could not hear me at all, that he appeared to have gone deaf, signalling his impairment not with confusion and effort but with blank stares, and I knew that he had been pushed even further into himself.

ar wax. That's all it was. The steady build-up of impacted
wax in his ear canals after weeks without attention, one of
those chronic conditions I'd forgotten he shared with
other members of his family, looked after routinely and easily
when he was healthy but sneaking behind the glittering stars of
this horror show for a place in the lowly chorus line upstage and
now stepping forward to steal a bow. So I laughed when the nurse
examining his ears announced the probable cause of his apparent
deafness, relieved by its benign familiarity, and she walked warily
around me as she went off to place an order for the drops that
might soften and release the blockage.

Lung failure, a serious infection, a heart attack, a stroke, kid-
ney malfunction, two bedsores, undiagnosed internal bleeding
and evidence of nerve damage that may or may not have been
caused by a stroke but so extensive that he could not move any
part of his body without pain, could not even scratch an ear,
never mind clean it. A tracheotomy that rendered him incapable
of speech. A tube to feed him from cans of beige liquid dumped
into a bag, another tube to drain his bladder into a discreet bedside container. Wired to monitors that constantly reported his

temperature, heart rate, blood pressure, respiration and other evidence that gathered to announce that he was still alive. A pale and diminutive version of himself, forty pounds lighter than he was before admission and always slim anyway, even his skin sloughing off onto his sheets, and I was laughing at the absurdity of having to shout at him simply because he was deafened by some sticky discharge from his cerumen glands that could normally be tidied efficiently at home were he able to even move his hands, which he could not.

The drops didn't seem to work. Days later, his hearing remained diminished and nursing staff could attempt nothing more aggressive to expel the wax until he was stronger. As an alternative to bellowing, never encouraged in a place where patients are always close to death, it fell to the alphabet card to be our means of communication.

The alphabet card is a profoundly stupid idea that must have been invented by someone with absolutely no understanding of hearing loss and its emotional impact on people whose bodies have already been trampled, and it is routinely used in hospitals to extract responses from conscious patients unable to converse. A nurse holds the card in full view of the patient and points to large printed letters, roaming back and forth with a finger through the alphabet until the right combination of letters produces the patient's intended word, a tedious exercise reminiscent of a Ouija board, with a trolling finger instead of a planchette. P-A-I-N — where? — L-E- — no, that's not it — S-H-O-U-L-D-E-R? — can take up to ten minutes to achieve, the process stepped along by the patient's nods or head shakes at each indicated letter. It is touted as a serious communication aid but in use it resembles the silliest of party games, and it even draws cheers when the campaign for the right word is successful. The patient is the only one not joining the celebration, faced with a clumsy and frustrating device made more ridiculous by its presence in a modern system that bristles with technological wizardry and that is proud of its progressive care.

Marg soon grew impatient with this. Mary's daughter, she was a frequent visitor and she decided there had to be more expedient means of eliciting answers from her uncle than a large card that forced a choice of twenty-six letters in organized combination. She arrived one day with her own solution: a list of basic questions for him, neatly printed out in large type that acknowledged the temporary absence of his glasses, all crafted to make him more comfortable. She held it before him:

PAIN?

WHERE?

IS BEDSORE HURTING?

HAD A BM?

WANT YOUR LEGS MOVED?

WANT YOUR ARMS MOVED?

WANT A BACK RUB?

It was primitive, but it helped for a few days, Jim responding with nods or headshakes. Yet I sensed there were things he wanted to say, troubling things lurking behind the wall of his pain, so I went to Donna Occhipinti, the unit's social worker and the kindly guide for families struggling to navigate a terrifying landscape. She was bright, energetic and efficient and listened to patients and families with complete attention and she was hearing me now asking if, I knew it sounded odd, but asking if the hospital had anyone who could read lips and she did not pause. "I think I know just the right person," she said. Next day she turned up at Jim's bedside with a woman in tow, a volunteer with other duties who happened to be completely deaf and who read lips, a kind woman who leaned in close to Jim's face and immediately frightened him into stony retreat with the force of her good-hearted zeal to help.

After that, some of us took turns trying to read his lips, but it was an uneven crusade. Mary could be adept at it one day and then back off in disappointment when she tried it the next. Marg would be rolling along, drawing him out as he struggled to form words, the two of them in comfortable exchange, then stumble over a phrase, unable to recover the thread. I took several runs at it, confident that anyone who had looked at those lips every morning for thirty years should be able to decipher their movements, and always failed miserably and always with a new respect for the skill. Some of the nurses were pretty good at it, Linda the Ken Follett fan better than most. She would be called from her own patient when Jim was agitated and tense, when it was obvious he had something urgent to communicate, and she could usually figure it out.

Then Al and Shirley made one of their regular visits, and Shirley fussed a little over Jim, straightening sheets, organizing his pillow, patting him on the hand, quietly praying for him as she bustled around, her natural instincts to comfort him, to somehow make all of his panic vanish by mustering devout and fierce determination, all on full and magnificent display, and Al was leaning over him, wrinkling his brow in concentration, studying his brother's lips, working to understand him, making this a project and assessing its challenges, and he suddenly stood up and turned to me. "I've got an idea," he said. "I'll call you later from home."

THIRTY

"Have you met Niki Garvey? She's offered to help."
Al asked the question without preamble when I
answered the phone that evening. Who? "Fred and
Theresa's granddaughter," he prompted. Well, now. Let me think.

Got it. Theresa is one of Shirley's older sisters. She married
Fred Garvey and their son is Niki's father. Niki had become the
subject of family lore. She was born with a serious hearing impairment but became so skilled at reading lips as a very young child
that it was years before her parents were aware there was anything unusual about her.

She arrived at Trillium with Al the following Sunday morning,
a striking woman in her mid-twenties, nervously clutching a cardboard cup of takeout coffee in the corridor outside ICU. It wasn't
until later that I learned she'd been in a serious car accident the
day before. She was uninjured but still shaken, and refused to
back out of her commitment to be here. We spent a few minutes
talking about Jim and his illness. I told her about everyone's efforts
to read his lips, about brief moments of success followed by long
gaps, about the foolish alphabet card and Marg's printed questions that helped and the very sympathetic volunteer who had

only succeeded in frustrating him, and she seemed to read my lips with ease, even when my head was slightly turned. "Let's see what happens," she said.

We all entered Jim's room and Al and I stood back, trying to stay out of her way while she approached him.

She greeted Jim, leaning toward him slightly so that she could see his lips in the dimness of the room. Her voice was soft and we could not hear what she said but we could pick up from her tone that it was kind and respectful. Jim looked at her and shook his head. She smiled and stepped back and waited, gazing out the window. She approached again a minute later and said something else to him and we saw his lips form a few words that only she could understand and once again she stepped away, this time to the doorway, gesturing us outside with her.

"He's afraid," she said. "He doesn't recognize me. He doesn't know why I'm here. Do you want me to continue?" Al and I looked at each other. "Please," I said.

We all entered the room again, Al and I standing back near the door. This time, he seemed more relaxed as she pulled a chair over to the bed, sitting close to him, then leaning into him, her face inches from his, and she spoke to him again, her voice too low for us to hear. Surprisingly, he seemed to understand her because he nodded in obvious response to something she asked. She waited a moment, then stood up and drifted in our direction. She said nothing to us. Instead, she looked over her shoulder at him and smiled. She waited a moment and returned to him, sitting again, placing her hand on the bed close to his but not wanting to presume by touching him. Al and I stared in wonder as he began to mouth words at her. We couldn't understand him but we could see he was agitated by the way his lips moved, and she listened with her eyes, undeterred by the respirator tube in his mouth, then leaned close to his ear, gently persuading him to continue and when he finally stopped some minutes later she said something brief to him and touched his hand and rose and smiled and left.

In the hall outside ICU, I was connected to Jim's present truths through Niki, as he told her, told me through her, about the constant pain that made any comfort an impossibility and about the fear and not knowing where he was or why, his last memories a phone conversation with a friend and then watching TV before he was suddenly racked with vomiting later that night. He did not remember anything since, remembered nothing of the first ambulance ride or the second one or the third, only knew that things happened and people were wisps in and out of his vision but not connecting any of it together into meaningful sequence. He knew he could not speak and most of the time he could not hear anything except shouts and he knew about the tubes linked to him but not why they were there or why his life was now this bed from which he could not flee, in which he could not even move, every effort overpowered. He was certain that all was desolation around him, that I had lost our home, that we had lost everything and I had sold his family keepsakes in order to survive, the 1919 gold medal that his mother had won for art and his father's pocket watch, not his railway watch but the fancy older one for special occasions. He believed that I was living in our car somewhere, that Hope had died and he mourned her loss, his heart broken because he would never see her again, that Bron and Murray had both died, that somehow this catastrophe had radiated out in waves from his failed body to assail and contaminate the lives of everyone he cared about. He felt guilty because it seemed I was there all the time and he had concluded that I had no place else to go but he was lonesome for me and he could not stop himself from wanting me there.

I hugged Niki and thanked her, hoping that some day she would realize what she had done to help his mending begin. She had touched him as no one else had, except for Betty at Mount Sinai when the tracheotomy was imminent.

After she and Al left, I found a corner and wept over the detritus of his suffering, all the harrowing things he had not been able to shed until now. I wiped my eyes and returned to his room and dragged the chair Niki used back to its place close to him, reaching for his hand, feeling him try to return the squeeze, pressure as light as an infant's clasp, and I was almost giddy when I began assuring him that Hope was alive and thriving and Bron and Murray were well and I was not living in the car and the house was very dusty but still ours, said it must resemble a time capsule because nothing had been moved or altered since he had left, raising my voice to be heard by him and not caring whether anyone else overheard. I told him I was here a lot because I wanted to be here a lot and the clothes I were wearing were the same ones I wore yesterday and the day before and last week and maybe that's why he thought we no longer had a home but they were clean and I couldn't be bothered selecting anything different until these were in rags because I didn't give a damn how I looked as long as I could keep coming here, keep being here with him, because that had become more important than anything else. I told him he was safe here, protected from harm, and this was Trillium Health Centre, that's right, the big hospital west of us, and they know what they're doing. I told him I realized it would take a while for all of this to sink in, for the nightmares to fade and drop away, but they would, they would, and for the first time his mouth formed the smallest of smiles.

A couple of days later, I intercepted an intensivist bustling between cases, one of the friendlier and more approachable clinicians, and raised the feasibility of adding a lip reader to the unit's resources, someone who could be on call for other terrified patients like Jim who have things they yearn to say but can't. I was still dazzled by Niki's transforming impact, and knew a doctor would have some influence and might carry the idea forward. I anticipated his willing support for something so obviously beneficial and figured he would appreciate that healing is more than the clinical restoration of bodies to their basic function.

"No need," he said, dismissively. "I'm a pretty good lip reader myself but I've found most ICU patients have nothing useful or important to say anyway." With that, he was gone, wrapped in his arrogant assumptions, leaving me to wish that he wouldn't have to be in Jim's dark place before he knew just how callous and disdainful he had been. Leaving me to wish that he would be hurled into Jim's dark place so that he would know just how callous and disdainful he had been. Leaving me to abandon those two clashing and unproductive impulses, a war of self-righteous opponents, and wonder instead at a bright and caring specialist whose first priority was to prolong survival but who apparently didn't understand that every aching and battered soul in his charge first hungers for release from overwhelming fright. *Hear the afflicted, then heal them.* Niki had helped ease Jim out of his darkness simply by listening, by connecting to him. This doctor would comprehend and value the legacy of her gift or not, and in his own time. No matter. It was enough for now to witness the pale but unmistakable flickers of returning light in Jim's eyes.

I had a photo to show him, a photo of his beloved Hope, posing demurely on our living room rug for the camera, with the pitted moonscape of her geriatric nose prominent in the frame and the compromised rear leg she had injured years before now extended out for comfort, her milky eyes disclosing a resigned acceptance of the human vacancy in her life. I held the photo close to him so that he could focus, reminiscing about a dog who came home with us from the Toronto Humane Society, no longer young even then, given three months to live, we were told, because the cancer she had was certain to spread rapidly, but not cooperating one bit with the solemn predictions in the six years since by surviving on some mysterious alliance of curiosity and determination. "I took this picture a couple of days ago," I said, assuring him again that she was eating well and enjoying her walks. He squinted at Hope, the look on his face embracing her and all the familiar terrain of our living room beneath and behind her and he nodded, clearly longing for her and for us as we were, a tear escaping from one eye.

I put the new photo together with the others that had magically survived the hasty transfer from Mount Sinai, then presented the collected group to him, holding them up one by one, Al, Shirley, Mary, John, Kathy, him, Hope and me, all taken in our home, showing the walls and the staircase in the background, sensing the will of his spirit to move toward the images, to who he really was and what he was part of and wanted to be part of again, some of the adhesive of his life finally present again.

THIRTY-ONE

ext day, I showed up in a different sweater and jeans, strolling around his bed in an improvised fashion show, knowing it was a sweater he liked, painting his vista different colours with it, hoping show-and-tell would confirm I wasn't living in a car. He looked at the old sweater, a bright woolly thing with obvious pulls and pills, and he raised his eyebrows. That was his only comment.

Sometimes I could successfully read his lips when he had something he urgently wanted to communicate, hoping I could ease the overriding steadiness of his discomfort. His requests were simple: move my legs, move the pillow, move a hand or an arm, tell the nurse I need something for pain. The nurses were administering scheduled doses of morphine, and had been since shortly after his return from Mount Sinai. He was fully conscious by now, fully aware of his pain. I would always report his need for relief to the nurses and sometimes had to tell him he wasn't due for a dose yet. He could move his fingers but that became impossible if the hand was covered with a sheet. He was capable of a single hand squeeze but it would be half an hour before he could summon the strength to repeat it.

It became important to raise him so that blood could start to flow vertically for a change and battered lungs could get used to working right side up again. But simply moving him more than an inch on the bed caused such obvious misery that nurses resisted anything aggressive. Even Mira was cautious, a veteran physiotherapist who coaxed small hand and foot movements from him while she played droning country and western music on a small portable radio that she carried around with her and that was intended to inspire her patients. Achy-breaky music for achy broken bodies. She hummed along with the music while she worked, cheerfully ignoring silent pleas from Jim, not hurting him but pushing him to his narrow limits, achieving gains that could be measured only in centimetres.

Ten days after his arrival back at Trillium, Linda and two other nurses teamed with Mira and shunted his bed around a corner to one of the few rooms in the unit with a ceiling hoist, a room that was temporarily vacant while its usual occupant was away for extensive tests. Linda and Mira took charge of the project. I watched closely as they planned and discussed just the right way to ease Jim from his bed and over to the chair padded with pillows that waited to one side.

Linda would call the moves while the others carefully placed a sling under him, a sling with formed sides and back that would hold him in a sitting position for the transfer. Mira's job was to monitor his breathing and blood pressure through the project. "Okay," said Linda, "we'll raise him on one side. That's it." Mira reached for the sling. "Let's see if we can work it underneath him." Linda was mindful of his tailbone bedsore. "Careful, everybody. Really slow," she said. "Now up to the shoulders for the rest of it. See if we can centre him. Make sure he's sitting fully in it.

Good. Okay, Jim?" She looked at him and seemed satisfied. The other two nurses held him upright. Mira attached the cables from the ceiling motor to each side of the sling, testing their security. All of this had taken about ten minutes. Linda then stepped back and reached for a boxy device with buttons, pressed one and Jim began to ascend slowly from the bed, then pressed another which guided the sling carrying him along a rail to a point where it rested a few feet above the waiting chair, his legs dangling beneath him. She pressed a button once more, and the sling lowered slowly toward the chair, a nurse moving it precisely under him so that his legs cleared the forward edge of the chair seat and he was settled into it.

He remained in the chair for nearly an hour, glaring at Mira who stayed to watch for signs of physical distress. I could tell he was miserable, hating every minute of this ordeal, struggling to fight his profound physical weakness and stay upright, thinking vengeful thoughts that thankfully remained private, his body goaded into improved cardiovascular repair. I sat beside him, pretending I didn't see his imploring looks but fretting until he was safely back in bed again.

A couple of days later, Mary and John came to visit and all three of us were with him when two male nurses entered and declared that they were going to remove him from his bed for some upright time in a chair, a procedure decreed by the doctor on duty that day. One of them was a muscular jock who faced the challenge like a football player ready for a scrum. While we watched, they proceeded to place a sheet under Jim and then to raise him slightly off the bed with it. His face was contorted. They were focused completely on their goal, the chair, were oblivious to Jim's visible discomfort while they worked. When I could tolerate no more of his silent anguish, his face starting to remind me of Munch's *The Scream*, I hollered at them to stop. They both looked at me in shock, still holding him above the bed but frozen in position.

"Can't you see he's in pain?" I demanded. "Look, Mira and Linda worked out all the moves to get him out of bed a couple of days ago. They used a sling and a ceiling hoist. Check his chart. Maybe they left some notes, some guidelines. This is not working!" Both looked nonplussed, uncertain how to proceed. Then, one nodded to the other and they lowered him back into the bed. His sigh was audible.

"Patrick, you're interfering. They know what they're doing," said Mary in a sharp voice that left two large and bewildered nurses standing like guards on each side of the bed.

I went over to her, straining to keep a lid on my fury, leaned into her face and spoke as quietly as I could. "They don't know what they're doing," I said, my jaw clenched. "If you've got a problem with me, let's take it outside. Not here, not now." Forty years as a nurse and she had broken one of those unwritten but inviolable hospital rules: you don't argue in front of a patient. Ever. I knew it by instinct. She should have known it by training.

"Well, he has to learn that pain is part of recovery," she snapped. "That's reality. You can't protect him from everything." She shook her head: "Sometimes I just want to slug you." At that moment I would gladly have taken a swipe at her and said so, drawing a look from John that said go ahead and try, and drawing a retaliation from Mary: "Just remember. I hit back."

Damn, I was angry. Angry at the two nurses for being so clumsy and offhand, angry at Mary for her trusting deference to them, to their inept and insensitive blundering, angry because I believed she feared they would retaliate and that Jim would pay for my defiance when we were absent, angry that no one in the room seemed to value my continuous and watchful presence in his care, vigilance that made me a useful link between one shift and the next. I looked at Jim and he mouthed my name in an effort to calm me. The nurses gently organized him back into his bed, and left, probably to mutter between themselves about annoying civilians who get in the way of unpleasant but essential therapy.

Mary and I glared at each other, saying nothing more, and then she and John left. I found them later in the waiting room and Mary and I made a peace of sorts, both of us acknowledging that we each had his best interests at heart but now tacitly determined to circle each other even more cautiously. We are so different, I thought. How can two people who care so much about the same person be so different?

Several days later, she and John were visiting again after they had taken their grandson on a ski trip. I watched Jim's eyes waver as she flashed photo after photo of snow banks and ski slopes and mountains past him. Then she apparently felt it was important to let him know how close to death he had come and how much he had improved since. "You have no idea how sick you were," she declared, by way of suggesting he might want to consider being grateful for his improvement.

After she and John left to meet Marg in the hospital lobby and we were alone, he struggled to communicate that he wasn't at all interested in hearing about his progress back from near death. "It doesn't change anything," he mouthed, his lips forming the words laboriously. I understood what he meant. He knew only the present, knew only that he hurt all over. Nothing else mattered.

I wanted to convey to Mary that it was unwise to talk about

the track of his illness, that it was not useful for him to hear how sick he had been, but I knew she would resist that advice from me. So I enlisted Donna Occhipinti, the unit's social worker, and explained the dilemma of two people who loved him and who kept butting heads. I told her that Mary would likely rebuff anything I suggested, that she would be dismissive of anything I might propose because I was not among the trained experts in charge of his care.

What I didn't share with her was that I also believed Mary still remained uneasy with the intimacy of our relationship, that she would not have challenged the spouses of her other siblings, would have allowed them their right to advocate for their partners as I had for him the day the nurses tried to move him. When Mary and John returned with Marg, Donna discreetly drew Mary into a side room for a private chat.

When she came back, she whispered an announcement: "Donna thinks we should concentrate on the present and the future when we talk to Jim."

According to Donna, said Mary, Jim did not want to hear how sick he had been. "It won't make him feel any better to know that he nearly died. Why don't we all agree we'll only talk about the present, where he is right now, and help him focus on recovery." I joined Marg and John in nods of docile agreement and said to Mary, "That sounds like a good idea. Let's try it." Feeling devious. Feeling victorious. Feeling that he had finally been handed back some control of his life.

THIRTY-TWO

There is a brawny trash bin to one side of Trillium's main entrance and I stall beside it after parking the car. I am weary and despondent, not yet primed for the long hours when I have to be buoyant with Jim, not wanting any of it. This is late afternoon but at any time of the day, people can be found near the bin with their cigarettes or cell phones, occasionally occupied with both at the same time, some standing with bags and plants and stuffed toys while they wait for transportation home, others walking back and forth in obvious distress, coping privately with troubling news, glancing mournfully at strangers. I look at my half-smoked cigarette and stub it vigorously in the large ashtray at the top of the bin, annoyed that the habit still clings but grateful for its companionship.

As with most modern hospitals, the Trillium lobby bows to commercial exigencies, with a Tim Hortons coffee shop, a gift shop that promises proceeds to the hospital, a drug store and a convenience store, all under a ceiling that is oppressively low. Visitors move differently here than they did at Mount Sinai. They are not brisk and purposeful. For the most part, they amble along deferentially, in step with each other like members of a tour group, and many of them arrive or leave in minivans, another clue to the conservative culture of this suburban setting that seems far removed from the cosmopolitan buzz of the downtown hospital lobby only a few miles away. Usually impatient with their languid pace, I have learned by now to dash past them, already adept at navigating the tricky turns of a hospital that has been grafted with various wings and additions over the nearly fifty years of its life. I know the short cuts to Jim's bedside. But today I am in no hurry to get there.

Perhaps it's the vulnerability that comes with fatigue but today I feel freakishly out of place here, certain that intimate homosexual relationships are rare in this environment that visibly prizes conformity. I know that the sight of one middle-aged man closely tending another might mystify and perhaps entertain my fellow visitors. I don't want their lives, don't even seek their acceptance, but today I envy their effortless compliance with unspoken rules of behaviour. I know they would have sided with Mary when I took on the nurses who tried to move Jim, deferring without question to them as she had. I had been uppity, gay and uppity.

The hospital volunteers are mostly white, elderly and female. They comply with established order by decking themselves in matching coloured smocks that differentiate them from the white coats of higher institutional authority. They often set up tables next to the information desk on the perimeter of the waiting area, an atrium off the lobby that feels like a sudden escape back into daylight, swaths of white cloth filtering the glass dome high above. There they fundraise by selling hand-knitted goods like matching hat and scarf sets and outfits for babies and various doodads of questionable utility, in addition to well-thumbed used books that run to the romantic in theme.

Behind them sit those who actually use the waiting area to wait, staring impassively ahead or engaged in earnest discussions about things like appointments and test results and prognoses. From a distance, one wall resembles a war memorial, with rows of names that seem to be a bronze salute to fallen soldiers, but it is actually a list of hospital donors, and instead of differentiating the officer class from enlisted men its hierarchy is determined entirely by gratitude, the most generous thanked at the top, followed by less significant supporters who are listed in alphabetical order.

A huge work of art dominates another wall. It was created by British Columbia artist Joanna Staniszkis in Plexiglas, hand-dyed wool and silk. A plaque says it is a tribute to John Cameron Pallett, the local member of parliament who officially opened the hospital in 1958. His family were liberal benefactors.

In surreal colours that jolt the eye, whimsical images of birds, flowers, trees, a stream and a waterfall are intended to evoke memories of Pallett's early 20th century birthplace in Dixie, a bucolic village of white Protestant sensibilities once centred only blocks from the hospital but now long gone, the area now a prime destination for seekers of new computers and floor tiles.

Up close, the project's visual impact is almost psychedelic, what was once called a head trip, and both terms would likely have distasteful connotations for most of the ladies seated behind me with their knitting. But it recalls an early Jefferson Airplane song, the one about Alice and the white rabbit that haloed the summer of 1967, the Summer of Love. "Go ask Alice," I hum. "She's a head."

Turning and then looking at the ladies from a distance, I imagine unruffled lives that have progressed without chaotic interruption or reckless adventure, lives that have stood firm against calls for radical change, all of their mind-altering drugs always legal, even a little queasy with the modern notion that marijuana can serve a medicinal purpose, smoothly ordered and predictable daily routines sutured by husbands and children and now grandchildren, always confident with their fixed place on the planet, a tribalistic adherence to common values and beliefs reflected in their faces and in their casual banter with each other.

This labour draws them because they see it as both noble and satisfying, bound as they are by an unconcealed impulse to place doctors on an exalted level, with their church ministers and other social aristocracy. They are afraid of the people on gurneys and in wheelchairs because they remind them of their own mortality. They can smell death on others, we all can, as surely as carrion birds. But they are kind, understanding that each patient is always less fortunate than they are and therefore in need of comfort.

Still, there is a pulsing entrepreneurialism behind their benign smiles, with some of old Ontario's loyalty to the socially enriching possibilities of capitalism. The volunteer department owns the Tim Hortons across the corridor from their tables, long lines of customers always winding out from the counter and around the corner toward the ladies and their wares.

All profits from the successful franchise go to the hospital, to this place that mends bodies that have often been abused by their owners. As I idle over a frosted chocolate doughnut laden with artery-plugging cholesterol, I realize every tasty bite is helping to underwrite the salaries of people like cardiac surgeons and nutritionists on the Trillium payroll. I stifle a chuckle at the irony, and order another doughnut.

THIRTY-THREE

"Are you planning to share the jackpot with the rest of us?"

I scowled at the source of the voice, a grinning young guy waiting behind me at the hospital convenience store counter, between us a pretty little girl in a stroller who immediately defused my crankiness and made me feel sheepish for nearly vaulting into a crabby response.

The embarrassing chocolate smudge from the doughnuts was gone from the side of my mouth, thanks to the clerk who had discreetly mentioned it and then mimed rubbing it away, and I was buying our weekly lottery ticket, ready to head upstairs to Jim for the evening, playing by rote the same old numbers, a combination of our birthdates, both of us always feeling like suckers because the most we'd ever won was $20 yet fearing our numbers would come up the very week we declined to play. Besides, I could tell Jim I had a ticket for that night's draw, yet another mundane detail from his life to fasten to his consciousness.

Unsurprisingly, it doesn't sell cigarettes, but like every other convenience store, this one offers the customary mix of expedient basics for tired visitors leaving late who can endure no challenge more complex than opening a can and starting a microwave when they get home. I was growing particularly fond of Chef Boyardee Beef Ravioli by then, a dietary choice that would have appalled Jim if he had known about it. Don't ask, don't tell. At least I hadn't yet cultivated a yen for those chewy things shaped like twigs and stuck unprotected in cups on the counter, the ones that claim beefy origins but never disclose what desiccated part of the cow was harvested for their production. Hooves come to mind.

"How old is she?" I asked, looking down at the child dozing in her stroller. "Sixteen months," he answered, and we struck up a conversation, which always starts between hospital visitors with a question about the purpose of the visit, a search for community in a setting that does not encourage it among people who are not staff or volunteers. To judge from his cheerful mood, I figured he was here for an older friend or relative facing something fairly routine, maybe gallbladder surgery or hip replacement or something else that usually results in speedy discharges, the patients carrying still-fresh flowers home with them, and I begrudged him the easier life he obviously enjoyed.

"Her mother. My wife," he answered without altering his mood, eyes flicking from the child and then to the ceiling to signify upstairs somewhere. "She had a major stroke a week ago, her second. She's only thirty-one. They're starting to get a little movement but she can't speak yet. May never. They don't know. We come in every day, spend as much time as we can just sitting with her. I want her to be able to see her kid, even if she can't hold her. I don't want her to lose who we are, to think we have left her life. What about you?"

I gulped and wished him well but could only imagine the deep sorrow he masked for the sake of his child, glossed over the details of my own reason for being there, and left for the elevators, angry at myself for rushing to presumption, wondering whether my judgement of the volunteers might also have been too quick, too glib, wondering if I was so deeply entangled in our own crisis that no one else's could possibly be more terrible, pondering the astonishing ability of the human spirit to simply adapt and prevail through the worst of life, sometimes without surface fuss or disturbance, exiting the elevator, climbing the few steps to ICU and then abruptly back into occupancy of our own nasty corner.

Mary was his nurse that shift. She was from Cape Breton and she had a lot of the island's dry humour that would quickly come out to play when she felt she could break briefly from the firm and diligent attention she paid to patients. She was always methodical with Jim, scrunching up her face with intensity whenever she looked at him and occasionally muttering to herself about unfinished chores. She would sometimes leave suddenly and without explanation and disappear around a corner, returning a minute later with supplies or medications or an assessment device of some kind, ignoring me until she finished whatever she had to do.

But when she allowed herself to relax a little, we would have some good chats and this night she talked about her worrisome mother who lived alone back home, worrisome because she was nearly blind and rebuffed any talk of a nursing home, announcing to the family that she trusted her homecare nurse and that she was fine so they should stop hovering, and we agreed that old people need their independence but their children often pay a high price in fretful nights. I told her about meeting the young father with his child downstairs, a family fractured by a stroke with uncertain consequences, and how his story helped me gain some perspective on what we were enduring.

By then, I was practised at helping with some of the basic bedside tasks like dressing changes and bathing, doing nothing more complicated than handing over fresh pads or antiseptic or whatever a nurse would normally have to stretch for, feeling part of his care instead of excluded from it, always wearing the disposable gloves that came off with a declarative snap. Jim's bedsores continued to need careful attention, and I watched for signs of improvement during every dressing change, hoping to see the tiny evidence of pink tissue that signalled each wound's slow progress toward closing.

I was now able to shave him, using an electric razor from home that first had to be sanctioned by the hospital's electrical authorities even though it was battery-powered.

Sometimes I would simply stand by with verbal support for him while a nurse fished a long tube into the tracheotomy hole, extending it deep into his lungs to suction excess fluid that he couldn't expel on his own. I would join the nurses in encouraging him to cough every time he was being suctioned so that he could begin the work of clearing his lungs on his own. I always listened carefully for any burbling sound in his breathing, a signal that suction was needed, and occasionally alerted staff to the need for attention before they were aware of it. Jim would tolerate the procedure without fuss, signalling his discomfort only with widened eyes, and he would try to expedite things by attempting to cough, seldom a successful venture.

This night, it was a bowel movement that had to be tended to. Mary did most of the work. All I did was whisk away the soiled blue pad and make sure a replacement and extra washcloths were standing by. It was important to keep him clean because fecal matter could infect the bedsore site nearby.

When Jim was comfortable, Mary announced she had to check another patient whose own nurse was on break and I thought I'd slip away for a cigarette and told her so. She suddenly looked horrified and I thought for a moment it was a kind of mock horror, exaggerated disapproval of the act, because we had been bantering comfortably only a moment before, so I laughed but then suddenly realized she was very serious and her reaction bordered on outrage. "You're smoking?" she demanded to know. "After all the damage to his lungs, you're still smoking? Haven't you learned anything from this?"

I was silent, not knowing how to respond, feeling chastened, then angry, and I tapped the pack in my shirt pocket.

"When he comes home," I said, with pious resolve, "I'll be gone."

What? What did I just say? Did I actually say, when he comes home, I'll be gone? Mary had no reaction. I wasn't even sure she had heard the words themselves, only the intent she wanted to hear.

I started to sweat, and looked away. I wanted to correct myself, wanted to retract, but didn't, wanted to say to Mary, I meant the cigarettes, not me, the cigarettes will be gone but I won't, I'll be there when he comes home, but didn't, couldn't speak because I knew that I had released something unbidden from way down in my gut that was harsh but enthralling, that all the weeks of clamped-down ache and grief and exhaustion had suddenly bubbled over, and I realized that being gone was precisely what I wanted right then. I craved freedom from all of this, the shit and the oozing sores and the tubes and the twittering machines and the day after day of his pain and the smells and sounds of illness and debility. I was tired of the platitudes from strangers who then retreated to the tranquility of their own lives, desperate for transport to some other place where ebullient and untroubled people gather in sunny rooms to talk about books and music and movies and ideas and all the normal things that can lift days into buoyant flow from one to the next. When he came home, yes, I wanted to be gone away from him and from this, from its drudgery and its anguish and its desolate confinement. I saw nothing of the future but this, together and trapped, or that, apart and freed, both clear and divergent options. In that moment after Mary walked away, I chose apart. It seemed I had nothing to lose.

Later that night at home, the phone rang. It was my sister, one of her frequent check-in calls. Maryalice is an Ottawa teacher and we don't see each other often but we are good friends.

I told her about blurting out something repulsive that surfaced so swiftly, so forcefully, that it rattled my core with guilt. What did it mean? Was I out to prove something by stubborn adherence to his bedside? Was it just grandstanding, this long and visible attendance through his crisis — the gay partner determined to slay stereotypes by caring more dynamically than anyone else, slyly entertained by shocked reactions to the enduring length of our unconventional intimacy? Was I saying, step back from your bias, straight people, and witness real love and commitment? And did I really want to bail, finally defeated by the hardest part of it, the acidic wait for something to change, and feeling that nothing ever would because this was now us, as fully realized as we would ever be, frozen like characters in a museum tableau? At that point, I started to blubber, unable to continue, knowing I really did not want to desire escape but finding the idea seductive and thrilling, my voice finally trailing off into bleating little self-pitying whimpers that mortified me.

She paused reflectively before responding. "I think," she said carefully, "that it's very important to pick the right moving company. I hear North American Van Lines are pretty good." There was a long silence. Then I started to laugh, and she started to laugh, and soon we were both convulsed. She had understood the impulse, knew it was born in bone-deep weariness, my own yearning for relief from pain as sharp as his, and then she had bridged to the fundamental absurdity of the questions. She knew I would not leave him, and even found the idea amusing, knowing me better than I do. It became a running gag between us. Every time she called from then on, her opening question was the same: "How's the packing going?" But I ended our call that night still wavering in my fidelity, still entranced by saying "I could go" out loud.

The next day, he started to bleed. That stopped my infatuation with flight.

THIRTY-FOUR

I t was into the early evening, around six, and it had been a good day. I had arrived around noon. He seemed fairly comfortable, reacting to people around him more positively than usual. Michelle was his nurse, just back from a long vacation and meeting us for the first time. We chatted easily, she talking about her early experience as a Canadian nurse in a British hospital, finding the environment more formal and constrained there than here, and I, about the sudden onset of Jim's illness and the quality of his care, both of us expressing wonder at how he seemed to be coming slowly back despite the high odds against him.

I was about to leave for home when she reported he'd just had a bowel movement. I paused and offered to help with the task of cleaning him and she hesitated, first time with the eager partner, after all, but he seems to know the moves, so what the hell, and we approached his bed, at ease with each other, raising him as usual to his side, monitoring his comfort, a fresh blue pad ready. That's when we saw the blood spreading on the pad beneath him. I was so shocked I found myself wondering why they call it a blue pad because this side, the absorbent side, was always white, a blank canvas for the body's brown expulsions, but brushed this time with vivid and intensifying swipes of red.

She confirmed his blood pressure was okay so she ordered a quick check of his hemoglobin, and I remembered the same test at Mount Sinai, remembered that hemoglobin is a protein carried by red blood cells that picks up oxygen in the lungs and delivers it to tissue but had not had to fret about it since. Normal range for most male adults is 140 to 175 grams per litre, a standard of clinical measurement that meant nothing to me. All I knew from Michelle was that his hemoglobin had suddenly dropped below seventy, that it continued to drop, evidence that he continued to bleed from somewhere inside, that he might need a transfusion. She was having trouble masking her concern, an obvious tension underlying everything she said. I was having trouble not reaching for a phone and calling Norma back at Mount Sinai, saying, look, he's bleeding again. One more time, could I hear you tell me not to trouble my heart, that they can fix that? We could use a fix here.

Jim seemed immune to the fuss around him. Michelle had been joined by another nurse who confirmed her assessment. "Are you aware that you're bleeding?" I asked him. He nodded. He did not look frightened. He seemed to know that blood was leaving his body at a quick rate but he was apparently unalarmed by its scary implications. Good, I thought.

Michelle went off for advice and a specialist arrived an hour later to confirm the need for an immediate blood transfusion. She introduced herself as Dr. El-Ashry and drew me to one side. "We may need to investigate," she said, as kindly as she could, and I recalled exactly those words from weeks earlier at Mount Sinai. I knew I was being cautioned again, that the process could be risky and uncomfortable. Do they all draw their conditional phrasing from the same playbook? To her colleagues she would have said, "We may have to scope him."

Once he was stable, I went home to sleep. The phone rang early in the morning. It was Dr. El-Ashry. "We need to investigate," she said. "He's still bleeding and we need to know why."

"You mean you have to scope him." A statement, not a question. She hesitated. "Yes," she said.

An hour later, he was enduring both an endoscopy and a colonoscopy as the specialist probed his digestive and intestinal tracts for anything from ulcers to tumours, one device down his throat and then the other up his rectum, the only good thing about the ordeal its evidence that he was now strong enough to tolerate the kind of invasion considered very dangerous while he was still at Mount Sinai.

She found nothing outrageous, Dr. El-Ashry said, using phraseology that was amusingly familiar by now. "Nothing outrageous" might not be good news but it wasn't bad. She had found no lesions, ruptured blood vessels or polyps. No obvious reason for the bleeding. The only answer to the next question — "What's causing the bleeding then?" — was a vague suggestion that it might have been induced by the drugs he was on as well as his long ICU stay. "It sometimes happens," she said. Within a day or so, the bleeding stopped and did not resume, leading staff to announce that it had spontaneously resolved, more hospital-speak, this phrase meaning we don't know what the hell caused it but it isn't a problem anymore so we can move on to other things.

Michelle herself had moved on to another patient by then but returned for a visit a few days later, and she smiled at Jim. She was more relaxed and admitted to me her terrible fear of the steady bleeding all through that anxious night. "I thought I was going to lose him," she said. So had I, and I understood that he was exactly what I had to lose by fleeing from this, understood that I was back, understood that I had never left.

THIRTY-FIVE

"Hello," Jim said. His first spoken word to me in nearly seven weeks was a wheezy exhalation that left him triumphant but exhausted.

The campaign to restore his voice started several days after the bleeding crisis, on a snowy afternoon in early February when I walked into his room and found him surrounded by two nurses, a respiratory therapist and a diminutive woman who introduced herself as Diana. "That's Diana, like the late princess," she said, in a manner that told me she said it frequently, accentuating the syllables but without a hint of vanity or guile, using the association with a royal celebrity only to make sure everyone understood the correct pronunciation of her name. She was not a Diane or a Dinah.

"I'm a speech pathologist," she said. "My job is to help wean Jim away from his tracheotomy." She spoke with the kind of didactic precision normally associated with elocution teachers. In her presence, I always found myself unconsciously mimicking her, lunging for all the nuanced details in every word, slowing my speech to form sentences with methodical accuracy. It made for interesting chats, each of us stepping with premeditated caution through our questions and answers, bystanders waiting patiently while proper diction was honoured. It wasn't my intention to mock her vocal patterns. Instead, the impulse to speak carefully was a reflexive fallback to a long-ago Jesuit education. Mumbling had always been discouraged. All vowels and consonants were expected to be audibly in place. "You speak very clearly," she said approvingly. "Did you receive training as an actor?"

Then she said something that stunned me: "Can you stay? I want you here for this." Dozens of doctors and nurses had already looked after Jim. Most had tolerated and even condoned my presence in his care but few had actively encouraged it. And none had requested it, until Diana. "You're the person closest to Jim," she said. "You should be part of this. It's important." I did not speak very clearly as I thanked her, turning away to hide how moved I was.

The plan to bring back his voice involved a complicated series of checks and assessments, all gathering to assure he could take air safely from his lungs past the tracheotomy site, up and over his idled voice box into his upper throat and then to his mouth and nose and back down again, just like a person who can breathe and talk normally. He would still need mechanical support to breathe but the tracheotomy that had done most of the work until now, which had become a muzzling fixture in his universe, was scheduled for removal.

It wasn't just a matter of extracting the tube from his throat and closing the puncture, although that would be an obvious side-benefit. Before she could even temporarily disconnect the tracheotomy for a trial run, Diana had to make sure Jim's oxygen rate allowed him to breathe without distress, and that's why the respiratory therapist was there to monitor the collapse and expansion of damaged lungs. He had to demonstrate an ability to control his own secretions, to be able to cough, because success or failure was determined by the amount of gurgling that could be heard in his chest. He passed all these tests but there were more.

As with all her patients, Diana also looked for basic alertness in him. Did he respond to greetings? Was he aware of her presence? She looked for compliance. Did he understand what was happening, why she was there, and did he agree with the plan? She looked for proof that he was oriented. "What is your name? Do you know what day it is? Do you know where you are?" Jim regarded the banal questions with mild disdain, rolling his eyes at every one, but answered them anyway, nodding and mouthing cooperatively. Diana was pleased.

Could he speak, after such a long time of enforced silence? That was a question no one could answer yet. There were fears his larynx might have been scarred by the tube down his throat that preceded the tracheotomy for nearly three weeks, always a risk for patients forced for longer than a few days to rely on oxygen by mouth. Even if his voice had survived, there was no way of predicting he would sound like himself. Nothing would be certain before he actually attempted to speak, and the team's superficial cheer didn't fool me. They were all tense, and their unease showed in clipped sentences overlaid with fragile optimism. They didn't have recourse to the relieving banter of an operating room. The patient was fully conscious for this one.

Once the team was satisfied that he was ready for a trial, nasal prongs carrying oxygen were attached to his nose and the tracheotomy tube was lifted from the flanged hole that always reminded me of the air valve on an inflatable beach toy. Then Diana capped the flange with a gloved hand that held a small square of sterile gauze, a process called "corking" that dates from the early days of tracheotomies when all of the flanges were stainless steel, not some variation of disposable plastic. Back then, each one was sterilized between uses and each patient had a personal plug made of cork that could be popped in and out of the hole as progress toward permanent closure continued.

Through the brief initial trials, Diana would encourage sound of any kind, even moans that made me wince but that apparently signalled promising response from his vocal chords. The first noise he produced was an extended "U-u-u-h," followed by "A-a-a-y" and "A-h-h." There was no resonance. The noises sounded like escaping cries.

Next day, she escalated to vocalization, again removing the tube and covering the hole, this time encouraging him to draw up the air for simple words to his mouth, to give them as much volume as he could, an agreeable coach urging him to watch and copy, and she would mime the effort of lifting air from the lungs, arms moving up her body.

"One. Try it, Jim."

"Whaa ... whaa ... on."

"Good! Now, two. Bring the air up. Watch me, that's it. Two."

"D-o-o ..."

Diana nodded at me. "Perhaps you'd care to take a turn," she said. Perhaps I would, I thought, trying not to move too eagerly to the side of his bed opposite her.

"Let's go for three," I said, and he nodded. "Three," I repeated slowly, extending it, pulling my arms up my body in imitation of Diana. His rendition came out as a stretched "f-f-ree" while he looked at me and then at Diana. The sounds were hollow and unfixed, like the harmless hauntings of cartoon ghosts. He got as far as seven before shaking his head, ready for a break.

A few minutes later, the counting resumed, on and off for an hour before the tube was reinserted into the hole. All of these first attempts at vocalization had been croaks and gasps that seemed to satisfy Diana but left me wondering if he would ever speak normally again.

Next day, I pressed my own gloved finger with a sterile pad over the hole, tentatively at first, my hand shaking slightly, afraid of hurting him, hearing a brief suck of air from the hole, then increasing pressure to seal it, Diana watching closely, cheering me on, and I told him that I was corking him, if that was okay, adding for the amusement of the team that the only thing I had ever corked was an unfinished bottle of wine and he smiled and I knew he remembered that we never emptied a full bottle over dinner when it was just the two of us but always saved some for the next meal, a modest ritual connecting our days.

And promise me you won't be quiet in the morning, I thought.

Diana will sometimes encourage patients to say "I love you" as their first words to intimates, an accomplishment that almost always provokes tears on all sides, nurses included, and she is respectful of the moment's powerful emotional significance but remains detached from it, weighing the quality and strength of the voice delivering the words, assessing the words themselves as potential signs of physical restoration.

But Jim ignored her gentle suggestion to say "I love you," and waited for me to speak first. We just knew that we would not say that to each other then, although I said it every night before sleep, said it to the embracing stillness as I had every night of our life together, an important finish to the day, and in his absence from our intimacy finding comfort in believing that he was still beside me. Beside me, but not yet there.

"Hello," I said, prompting him, wondering if he could summon the air and muscle required to push out a reply, hoping for him that he would not fail. I waited. Seconds passed and then he seemed to stiffen. "Hello," he said in reply, extending the word until it sounded like a very distant shout from the other side of a mountain, sounding like him way out of sight but coming back to me, he was coming back to me.

He waited for a response, pleased with himself. I leaned in and said, "Do I know you?" — deliberately aping his nervous challenge to me the first night we met, the first words he said to me, going back across all the years to the fever of our uncertain newness, trying for a copy of his impatience back then but failing, blinking back tears instead, shutting out all others in this room from our private jest.

He smiled and then shook his head, a mock rebuff, and I sensed he was surprised and entertained by the old question, long a familiar tease by now, but he was incapable of any further struggle for conversation, and the tracheotomy was reconnected.

BUT ONLY UNTIL the next trial and the one after that, each one longer and more successful than the previous, and the testing process would stretch for days until there might come a time when the tube would leave permanently, a tentacle releasing another piece of his body back to him, letting him say hello to me, to himself, for himself.

Do I know you?

THIRTY-SIX

e didn't want to talk about us or home or family two days later when I briefly corked his tracheotomy with a gloved hand, getting good at it, and he spoke, his voice now gaining slightly in strength but still foreign, as though he were fighting a sore throat. He was agitated. He wanted to talk about morphine, how he needed it, how he loathed the needing of it.

At another time, Jim might have been tickled by the reminder that morphine is derived from a variety of the poppy, one of his favourite flowers. But not now when he was clearly distressed, struggling to communicate his anxiety about its daily shadow in his life.

Two worries emerged from him, each linked to the other. He was afraid of developing an addiction to the morphine he required for pain relief, and he had lost any sense of his own body behind the narcotic's soothing cover. He often delayed asking for it until he could tolerate the pain no longer, then felt embarrassed by his dependency on it, and told me so.

I was heartened by his push to rebuild a complete image of himself, his mind and body slowly reconnecting, but I didn't know what to say about the addiction part. All I knew was that morphine is an element of opium, which comes from the poppy, and my mind flashed on an image of Victorian opium dens, glassy-eyed and recumbent addicts murmuring languidly to each other. I cringed at the possibility that Jim might be trading one struggle for another.

I went off in search of advice, for something I could say that might pacify both of us, and huddled with a small group of ICU nurses who happened to be at the desk. Was he in danger of becoming an addict? They all shook their heads, and one nurse claimed there's solid medical evidence that says patients in need of morphine for severe pain rarely develop addictions if they don't already have a history of substance abuse. Another nurse cited a massive Boston study of nearly 12,000 patients who were administered morphine while in hospital. "Only four were identified as addicts later on," she said. "Jim has no history of drug abuse, no predisposition to addiction. The morphine he gets goes right to pain relief. It doesn't give him a rush or a high. It doesn't give him any of the euphoria addicts are chasing. It just eases his pain."

Oddly, that kind of plausible conclusion, backed by serious study, hasn't eased fears of addiction among families and among clinicians who haven't had to treat acute pain. Maybe they've been spooked by too many horror stories, images of too many casualties, in a culture locked in endless warfare with illegal drugs. It seems fear of addiction has become addictive itself, leading pain specialists to argue that some patients are suffering needlessly because they aren't being administered appropriate doses of morphine.

But what about the other part, his urge to withdraw from morphine so he could begin to integrate back into himself, pain and all? "That's normal, and it's actually a sign he's getting better, so you're right about that. But tell him he's going to need it for a while longer. He doesn't have to be a tough guy. He doesn't have to prove anything. Try and assure him there will come a day when he won't need it. Try and give him some hope if you can."

I couldn't. I returned to him, feeling optimistic, carrying everything I'd learned, eager to help him into peace with his need, and I failed.

"All I know is this," he said after a minute, in a voice so low I had to ask him to repeat himself, to make sure I heard correctly. "This is all I know." He was louder this time, his voice still wispy but clearer. I understood what he meant. All he knew was a present filled with discomfort, knew nothing on the other side of it, and I could not move him from that position. He was not being obstinate. He simply saw no future, no escape from a prison defined by pain, and all of the cheery banalities and scientific studies wouldn't change that. Even the slow but steady return of his voice only allowed him to express out loud that he still felt ensnared and incomplete.

I sensed he was starting to slide into depression, an old enemy, and made him promise he would let me know if that was happening and if he needed help. He agreed. Next day I asked him again and this time he nodded, angry at his need for help, feeling weak and incapable of self-repair. The unit summoned a hospital psychiatrist, aptly named Dr. Head, who prescribed a mild tranquilizer. A psychologist then spent some time with Jim, a considerate man who listened and tried to take him away from this and into his forgotten daily pleasures again, encouraging him to consider the possibility of a normal life again, a goal which seemed foolishly distant, to him and to me.

Mira the physiotherapist continued to make daily appearances, lugging her portable radio with its rasping country music and planting it beside her while she persuaded imperceptible movements from his atrophied muscles. One irritating tune that involved a dog and a truck prompted her to announce that it had worked wonders on an elderly woman in the therapy whirlpool downstairs. "That song had her dancing in the water," she said with obvious glee, cranking up the volume in deference to his still-reduced hearing. "We'll soon have you dancing just like her." Jim grimaced when Mira wasn't looking, no doubt contemplating a fate that would fast-forward him into decrepit old age, life's meaning reduced to skinny white legs that quivered and twitched underwater in time with a twangy guitar.

Family members drifted in and out, solicitous and steady in their endurance, speaking with exaggerated clarity so he could understand them, even though his hearing was gradually starting to improve from the daily administering of drops. By now, his tracheotomy was corked much of the time with a removable plastic button, and he was starting to complete sentences. Mary brought coffee and sandwiches that she shared with everyone, and she once wondered aloud in his room whether he was feeling left out because he was still unable to swallow and still took his nourishment through a tube. But he had no interest in food, and said so. He had forgotten what anything tasted like. He had forgotten, and didn't care.

He also had no interest in visitors except family, turning me into an unpopular gatekeeper with friends who called and pleaded to see him, some in tears. Not yet, I would tell them as gently as I could but not sharing with them his emphatic resistance to anyone requiring effort or engagement.

As the days passed, I could also see that he was slowly becoming institutionalized, his reactions blunted under the weight of scheduled routine, and he would meekly cooperate with every procedure performed by the nurses, surrendering any final traces of dignity to probes and pats from strangers, their muttered apologies only a formality, no doubt pleasing some of them with his compliance. All privacy gone, now not uniquely himself anymore.

I knew it would take something startling and unpredicted to jog him from his angst, something to signal motion and change, and it occurred the afternoon I came walking into his room, expecting to find him supine and morose as usual, ready to read quietly at his side, ready to just be there, but instead he was sitting in bed, a bunch of pillows behind him, supporting him, his tracheotomy corked with the little plastic button, the bed beneath him stripped to the inflatable air mattress that relieved pressure on his bedsore, his chart propped against the bed rail beside him, a nurse named Tara feeding him ice chips like a court attendant.

I frowned at Tara, making no effort to conceal my alarm. "What's going on? Are you moving him to another room? Is something wrong?"

"Everything's fine. He's being transferred out of ICU and onto a recovery floor. Med 4D," she said.

"Oh. A recovery floor. Med 4D. Right, got it. When?" I asked, still unable to reconcile his gloomy mood of the days before with any prospect of recovery.

"Right now. We're just waiting for the word to go."

I flapped and sputtered about no warning and the tyranny of hospital clocks that ticked to unexplained schedules, another sudden spin like the trip from Mount Sinai to here, another phantom hand dialling up the turbulence, knowing it was a move forward and yet not joyous but irrationally thrown by the surprise. This was supposed to be good news, and I was angry at myself that I could not turn to it.

"Patrick?" I heard the wheeze and looked down at Jim, composed and apparently comfortable. He tried to reach for my hand. "I need you to relax," he said.

"I'm relaxed, I'm fine," I insisted, taking his hand, and he smiled at the childish lie. He's not ready for this, I thought. I'm not ready for this, I thought.

THIRTY-SEVEN

"*H*e's very sick." That had been Dr. Bill McMullen, sombre and troubled, those first hours long ago in Emergency.

"He's very sick." This was McMullen again, repeating himself eight weeks after that first morning, his tone still foreboding, but he was charged now with following the patient he'd tossed to ICU way back then, hefting Jim's hospital chart now, a volume in a large blue binder that had grown fatter and heavier than a big city phone book. He held up a dismissive hand. "No questions. I need to review this. Who did you say you are?" I almost laughed, but allowed him his ignorance.

He might not appreciate how absurd and patronizing he sounded when I asked for time with him, wanting to contribute, to make the point that I had never been a bystander in Jim's care. I had written myself in as a full partner. I was now a scrawny veteran of this battlefield. I had useful things to say.

How else would he know all that Jim had endured, all that we had endured together, always closely together, through all the bleak and stunting days since those first hours of chilling doubt? How would he know that I was more familiar with Jim's case now than he would be when he was finished reading about it? He might absorb the clinical case details from those endless chart entries before him, milestones like "failure to extubate" and "bleeding resolved" and "episodic seizures." But I also knew all the rest, could provide the defining personal texture of this journey, the apprehension and the dismay and the cautious hope underpinning all of the catalogued afflictions and remedies.

"Take your time," I said sharply to his retreating back, white coat snapping as he headed briskly for the nursing station to settle in for a long read. "It's *War and Peace*," I added. Meaning the voluminous bulk of his reading challenge. Meaning, doctor, it has been mostly war and some peace.

An hour earlier, Jim had been briskly transferred in his ICU bed to his next destination because a gurney wasn't available and the move had to happen too quickly to wait for one. Another patient had a pressing need for his vacant ICU room, and its bed was due back. But he could keep the special mattress, the one that inflated to relieve pressure on his bedsore.

Officially, the new unit was called Medical Recovery, two levels up from ICU on the fourth floor of D wing, but Trillium shorthand made it Med 4D and that's where three nurses and I wrestled the borrowed bed around a tight corner and into a cramped semi-private room, already strained to its limits by two beds, a flimsy curtain between them. At first, the ICU bed resisted all effort to place it next to the new one so he could be eased from one to the other. It behaved like an obstructed bumper car, fighting us, rubber fenders colliding with tables and IV poles. The mattress with its tiny built-in electric pump was already starting to lose air, sighing into gradual collapse, Jim sinking into its folds, and frightened. The large family surrounding the man in the room's second bed tucked themselves into corners and hugged walls, trying to stay out of the way.

We jockeyed the ICU bed so that one was adjacent to the other, grunting and muttering, air continuing to leak from the disconnected mattress, a nurse whose tag said she was Heather leading us through an awkward shuffle of reverses and forwards, three colleagues and a stranger suddenly thrown together for a common goal. Heather decided he should be transferred to his new bed right on his mattress, so we each took a corner, ready to lift.

"On your count?" asked Heather, looking across at me, and I knew the invitation was a test. I knew I was an ongoing presence in Jim's chart, knew it from ICU nurses seeing him for the first time and then greeting me like the familiar appendage that I had become. No doubt Heather had already heard about me, word passing informally from one unit to another, nurses chatting over lunch in the cafeteria about the two gay guys in ICU, and she wanted my measure: Will this one be helpful or annoying? Families can be annoying. Will he get in the way? Many do. Will he want to take charge? Some do.

"No," I said. "On your count." Heather simply examined my face for a moment, then counted. On three, we settled him into his new bed, a nurse and I skittering backwards across it to keep the transition smooth, our backsides billowing the privacy curtain. I heard a gasp of alarm from the patient on the other side. The ICU bed was quickly rolled back into the hall, ready for return. The mattress under Jim was plugged into the wall and immediately began to draw air again, this time inhaling instead of expelling, a discreet but reassuring hiss, and I watched him rise slowly like Lazarus from the sags and folds. We had arrived. I sat with him, saying nothing, both of us trying not to overhear the nervous voices on the other side of the curtain. Down the hall, McMullen continued to read.

THIRTY-EIGHT

he moon was in the seventh house and Jupiter was
something with Mars so something-something peace
and dawning of the age of Aquarius, age of Aquarius.
Aq-uar-i-us! Aq-uar-i-us! "Come on, Ted! Sing along with me!"

The tune seemed to be coming from the nursing station,
behind the front counter and out of sight of the elevator I was
stepping off, a woman's voice belting the old hit from *Hair* but
flattening the melody, pausing only to urge a duet, and I walked
over and peeked around the corner. An elderly man was dancing
with a much younger woman in a nurse's uniform, his open hospital gown playing peek-a-boo with puckered buttocks, a goofy grin
on his face. She paused and introduced him and herself. He was
Ted and she was Mabel and I watched them as she waltzed him
past me, past the counter and down the hall and into his room,
singing of sympathy and trust abounding. This is health care with
a difference, I thought.

It was the first morning after Jim's discharge from ICU. Later
I would learn about Ted's quirks and his tendency to drift into
patients' rooms any time of the day or night, simply to stare and
smile, or to loiter at the nursing station with no apparent purpose,

murmuring incoherently to the nurses there, his physical diagnosis never disclosed to the rest of us but something serious anyway, and with evidence of mild dementia in the way he benignly ignored boundaries, a lonely and innocuous refugee who was never very clear about anything except his love of music and dancing. Mabel also loved music and dancing, which she deemed beneficial to his serenity, and she became his unofficial guardian in the absence of any family and advised anyone pestered by Ted to shoo him away with a sharp word. "He means no harm," she would say defensively.

Mabel was one of the Med 4D nurses, in a 32-bed unit that was called a recovery floor but also housed patients like Ted, whose condition appeared to be chronic, whatever it was, and Jim's roommate, who was awaiting transfer to a cancer facility for further assessment, and now Jim himself, a bewildered new arrival with a prognosis that was still uncertain.

Tina was Mabel's boss, a quick, smart head nurse who never seemed to settle in one place but prowled the halls restlessly, even pacing while on the phone, twisting and unravelling its cord around her fingers while she spoke about patient conditions and medications and nursing assignments. There was an easy camaraderie among all the nurses, and most of them were swift to laugh, greeting family members with open-handed informality.

All except Nomita, who retained a secure distance from any jocularity. She was considered the unit's doyenne, an elegant senior presence in Med 4D's turbulent universe. As the daughter of a public health doctor in India, she had studied nursing in the early years after independence. Her training instilled the need for polite reserve around strangers, a possible legacy of the British Raj, and she was conditioned to rise whenever a doctor entered the room, to stand respectfully back and wait for instruction.

But several doctors told me they always listened carefully to what Nomita had to say about a patient. Her assessment skills were considered unerring.

For her, partners and families could be peripheral distractions. Jim liked and trusted her, despite her obvious discomfort with his occasional tears of frustration. In her world, men bore their pain stoically. She and I reached an amiable truce with each other, once she realized I wasn't there to second-guess her.

I found myself drawn close to all of these people as the days passed, to their steady compassion through twelve-hour shifts of grinding routine. Mabel fooled no one with her impulse to burst giddily into song. At heart, she was deadly serious about her patients. So were Catherine and Christine and Sundree and Helena and Yvonne and Cecilia and Pat and Belinda, and all the others I grew to know well because they saw Jim regularly, which meant they saw me regularly. Most of them accepted me as an unvarying presence, glad of an extra pair of hands for any everyday task. The only hint of any puzzle about the nature of gay relationships came one night when I wasn't there. A nurse attending Jim for the first time wondered who this Patrick was that she had heard so much about. "So. Is he your gigolo?" she apparently asked. Jim was still irate when he told me the following morning. I was amused. I liked the rakish tilt to the word.

Because he was still at high risk, he was moved to a private room a few days later, and it happened to be Valentine's Day so I brought some roses. A cliché, I knew, but the first flowers allowed close to him since admission.

That was also the day his tracheotomy was finally removed, no more corking trials needed, a smooth withdrawal of the flange, the puncture then dressed with a neat patch of gauze, nasal prongs in place to help him breathe. When we were alone, he could finally speak words that needed no prompting by Diana, no finger over the hole to test clinical volume and resonance, summoning not just air but his heart.

"I love you," he said.

THIRTY-NINE

*W*illie and Nah worked with him every day, the good cop/bad cop physiotherapy team. Their task was to restore Jim's shrunken core muscles, the ones that allowed him to hold himself upright and then to extend and reach without toppling over.

Nah was a tiny woman, Willie was a big man. Nah played bad cop, belying her size. Willie would first lift Jim so that he sat precariously on the edge of his bed. Then Nah would wheel a table in front of him, with a collection of bright plastic rings and poles scattered on its surface like toys. Jim would have to drop the rings over the poles, easy work for any child but he stretched and grunted with the effort. Sometimes, Nah would remove his glasses and put them a few feet away from him on the bed, forcing him to turn and reach for them, a major undertaking. Willie would be gentle and encouraging but Nah would be tough, pushing Jim to his limits, ignoring his glares and protests, cajoling wasted muscles into movement. Despite the ordeal, he began to look forward to their visits.

Once, I walked into his room after they'd left and he reached up absentmindedly to scratch his forehead, a familiar gesture that was part of his old fidgets and habits. But then he suddenly looked startled. "Did you see that?" he asked.

"See what?"

"This," he said, and reached up again to scratch. He looked delighted.

I had nearly missed a breakthrough. I smiled at him, sharing his pleasure. Until now, he had not been able to raise either arm more than a few inches. Willie and Nah were succeeding. His atrophied muscles were slowly healing.

When they left, Elise the occupational therapist would step in and help Jim kick-start some of the moves of a normal person in a normal life, if kneading clumps of Plasticine can be considered an everyday activity. The first time, he was presented with two clumps, one for each hand, but somehow managed to spread them all over himself and around him, rogue pieces escaping in all directions and adhering to every nearby surface with a tenacity that required a pause for serious clean-up.

Dinette was Elise's assistant, and she worked with his knees and feet and arms, teasing flex from rusty joints. He grew to like and trust her but then he suddenly developed clostridium difficile, abbreviated to C-Diff, a common and treatable hospital affliction that results in acute and unpredictable diarrhea. He saw it as a mortifying setback, an impediment to further exercise and therapy. "Dinette's due to come in," he said. "Tell her I'm not in the mood today. Don't tell her I can't stop shitting." His disappointment was obvious.

I intercepted her when she appeared at his door. "He's got C-Diff," I said, "and he's uncomfortable and embarrassed. Maybe another time?" Dinette looked past me at him. "Can I have a couple of minutes with him?" she asked.

When I returned to his room a while later, they were laughing together and talking and he was slowly bending his trembling knees up from the bed sheet. Later, he told me that Dinette had shared a piece of her own life, a serious car accident that had killed her young child and put her in a body cast for months. "She wasn't looking for sympathy," Jim said. "She just wanted to share something from her life." I was grateful to her. She had not made light of his C-Diff or his discomfort. She had simply dared to expose some of her own remembered pain and with that generosity had given him some perspective on his.

Bill McMullen appeared every morning, often announcing that he had trolled the internet the night before and found this or that illuminating piece of reputable information about Jim's condition. We were easier with each other now, and his dry humour was starting to emerge. Once, when I was on the other side of the bed, he suggested that Jim would probably be assessed by a physiatrist. "What's that?" I asked. McMullen looked pleased. "You don't know what a physiatrist is? That's a medical doctor who specializes in physiotherapy. Jim will need lots more of that down the road." I think he was pleased because he'd finally caught me on something I didn't know.

I became proficient at using the suction machine that drew bilious yellow discharge out of Jim's mouth, goo still surfacing from his lungs that he couldn't completely expel without help. Rick McRae, Mary's son, Jim's nephew, was a frequent visitor and the only member of his family comfortable with the suctioning task and we took turns when he was there. The old machine made a loud noise that abruptly halted all conversation and it collected its unpleasant harvest into a large glass vial, an accomplishment that always resulted in satisfied nods. Jim had changed Rick's diapers when he was an infant. Now Rick was busy tidying discharge from the other end of his uncle's body, the comical implications not lost on either of them.

"Turnabout is fair play," said Jim, glancing at the vial.

FORTY

The bedsores were healing, the one on his elbow much more quickly than the tailbone wound, which still gaped with a menace that could be unnerving. I was now skilled at assessing it, encouraged by Dr. Frank Rosenberg, a brusque but friendly dermatologist called in for regular assessments. The first time he appeared, I started to leave, by now accustomed to giving doctors the proprietary privacy with Jim that they all appeared to need, feeling extraneous but used to it.

"Come back here," said Rosenberg curtly over his shoulder. "I want you to see this." He pointed to an area of the wound. "Damn poor light in here. Gotta remember to carry a flashlight. Anyway, that area is healing. See that? Not just the pink granulation. I'm sure you know about that. But the pattern, look at the pattern. Thought for a while there he might need a skin graft. Nope. I think he's going to be all right. These things take a long time. Okay, you can dress it." The latter was said to Jim's nurse. Rosenberg nodded at me, and left.

Any time I saw something about the wound that puzzled me,

I would ask Tina to call Rosenberg. He would always show up within the hour.

I was learning that wounds seem to have a life of their own, charging ahead to heal and then suddenly pausing as though the effort has left them exhausted. It could be a baffling process to watch, and days would pass when there appeared to be no change at all.

There was one shift where a nurse I'd never seen before entered Jim's room to change the dressings. She accepted my assistance, and she cleaned the bedsore and changed the dressing with quick and gentle care, making no comment while she worked. I walked her to the hallway.

"Boy, that's some bedsore," she said when we were out of Jim's hearing.

"You should have seen it last week," I said, eager to reassure her. "There's a lot more pink granulation than there was. It's getting better." She blinked, clearly startled by an amateur's assessment. Then she smiled.

"Good to know," she said, and walked away.

I realized I was finally becoming acknowledged by staff as the continuity in his care, the linking personal resource between shifts, and it wasn't long before his nurses would ask me how he was doing. I was never thrown by a question that was commonly asked, and I understood their need to be aware of any change in his attitude or behaviour that might affect their clinical work.

An easy give-and-take developed. At one point, I thanked Tina for making me a partner in his care. "That's okay," she said. "We knew you weren't going away so we decided to put you to work." She could also ask me how he was doing, and I knew what she meant, and I would ask the same question later on, and she would know what I meant and I took to calling her every morning before coming in. She would tell me about the night he'd had, about his mood and energy level that day and about any test results, and I always knew what to expect when I arrived at the hospital, checking in with the nursing station once more before making the walk down the hall to his room, adjusting my anticipation, ready for whoever he was that day, ready to be wherever he was.

I often carried *The Wind in the Willows* and it was almost a good luck charm by now but I skimmed it silently while he dozed, finding its blameless pleasures oddly consoling but never daring again to read it to him as I had at Mount Sinai, still fearing a return of annoying tears. Once I asked him whether he remembered anything of those terrifying early days when he seemed to be slipping away. He was silent for a minute. Then he suddenly recalled a dream from that awful time, a happy image of the two of us relaxing together on a blanket in a field, me reading to him from a book. He didn't remember what I was reading but he remembered feeling content and peaceful under a sunny sky. His telling had a fence around it, as though all the rest of his dreams then were nightmares but this memory was not. This could rise now, and be enjoyed without fear or confrontation. I wept when he was finished but I did not tell him why. Ratty would understand.

WE HEARD A Code Blue call one evening, heard the distinct but neutral tones of a voice announcing the crisis, heard "Code Blue, Med 4D, Code Blue, Med 4D," heard rushing feet, heard the crash cart go clattering by his open door toward a room down the hall, an uncommon occurrence in a unit where no one was expected to need resuscitation. I waited a while, then left to stroll to the nursing station, finding familiar faces downcast, the outcome clear, knowing they would take the death of one of their patients personally, and I extended clumsy sympathy. Mabel and Nomita were both there. "She was fine just an hour ago," said Mabel. "She was stable when I looked in on her," said Nomita.

I was back in Jim's room for about thirty minutes when Nomita entered. This was a surprise because her shift was over. She should have been on her way home. Jim was awake and in a good mood. "He's doing so well," she said.

"We were just talking about food," I said. "I asked Jim if he was looking forward to eating an apple again. He loves apples, and one of these days he's going to be able to bite into one."

"One of the first things I had after we came to Canada was hot apple pie and ice cream in a restaurant on Yonge Street. I thought, I might not like this, hot and cold on the same plate. But it was delicious," she said, smiling at the memory.

"I bake a very good apple pie," said Jim. "When I get better I'll make you one. I'll even supply the ice cream."

"That would be nice," she said. "Good night." She turned toward the door and then back again. "He's doing so well."

It was some time after she left before I realized why she had come, why she needed to see life and healing, why she needed to see the other side of her work, righting the balance before going home.

Sometimes I stayed longer with him than I should have, fussing with the pillows under him so that he could rest with reasonable comfort on his tailbone bedsore, hating to leave, him hating my leaving, lying when I asked him whether I had the pillows just right, but both of us agreeing that it wasn't fair to an old dog with an uncertain bladder. One night I arrived home later than usual to find that Hope had peed, vomited and defecated on the kitchen floor, all three deposits placed strategically within inches of each other, something she had never done before, but voicing her protest now in the most effective way she knew.

Tina encouraged a therapeutic visit from Hope, dogs in hospitals no longer a big deal, something I thought Jim might enjoy. He shook his head. "I don't want her here. I don't want anything from home here, to make it feel like home. This is not home. This is only where I am for now." He was starting to see himself as a transient, someone just passing through this place, and I was glad.

FORTY-ONE

There are moments in every caregiver's life when all the wheels are turning, all at once, and it can be exhilarating. The hospital no longer feels like a faceless institution but becomes a generous and enlightened ally. Doctors and nurses banter easily with each other and with the willing caregiver, sharing smart information and ideas among themselves with the enthusiasm of a confident team. Those days seem to hum and soar with purpose.

On such a day I went sailing into Jim's room, shucking off my coat and tossing it on a chair as I approached him. Blood tests showed steady improvement. Heart rate was good. Blood pressure was sliding up into normal range. Lung function continued to return. He was moving more easily. He was recovering.

But I found him subdued and withdrawn, facing the window with the falling snow outside, and that was not surprising because the road to healing is never a straight line. I already knew his moods would swing from optimism to despondency as they do with every patient after a long hospital stay.

Catherine came in to change the dressing on his tailbone

bedsore and I helped her steady him on his side as usual, alert as usual to any change in the pathology of the wound, certain I would know what to look for, saw tiny pink signs of more new tissue, and smiled. Catherine leaned toward the wound. "It's coming along, isn't it," she said. "That's good." Jim was passive. "The bedsore's getting better," I said to him. There was no reaction.

After she left, I bustled around, topping up water jugs and replacing empty Kleenex boxes and organizing plants and flowers and cards, infused with the jovial energy of the committed and fulfilled. Finally, I relaxed in a chair beside him, blocking his view of the relentless white outside, and asked him how his day was going so far. He looked away from me. "I just want you to touch me," he said, his eyes suddenly filling with tears. "I just want you to be close."

Close? I thought I had been as close as anyone could be, through all these hard and fearsome weeks. But I realized I had never dared to touch him meaningfully, had not dared any kind of intimacy yet. I had not been repelled by him, ever, not by the clinical debris of this illness, the wounds, the diarrhea, the rickety physical limits and the husky and faltering voice — but I was still deeply afraid that I would somehow injure him further, assault him with a clumsy touch. He seemed so fragile, so vulnerable. I loved him more than anyone, would do all I could for him, thought I had done all I could for him, but I had not answered his hurting need for nearness, had not moved to reconnect us as we had been, for him a condition of his wholeness, for both of us the restoration of *us*.

So we sat and simply held hands, really held hands, and we talked.

"I feel broken," he said. "I feel like I will never be whole again."

You are broken, I thought. You are Humpty Dumpty after the fall, and all of these king's horses and king's men may fail to put you together again.

"That's not true," I said. "It'll take time but you're on your way back. Look at the progress you're making. I want you to know I'm in for this, all of it, the whole ride, no matter what it takes. Never forget that." His body was recovering. But his heart and spirit were scabbed. I struggled for a way to heal them.

Later, I organized the pillows under him, dimmed the lights in the room, kissed him good night and left the hospital convinced that I had been a good caregiver that day, there for him with comfort and assurance, efficiently interacting with the staff, enjoying accomplishment and the rightness of what I was doing, glad we had crossed some kind of gap between us, rode the parking garage elevator to my car, knowing the next phase of the journey had begun, and feeling excited about it.

I eased into the driver's seat and reached with the key to start the engine and stopped because I was suddenly crying, suddenly besieged by deep grief and pain and a sense of piercing loss, for that moment feeling as broken as he was by what had overtaken us. It was half an hour before I could move. But I remember being glad that I was alone.

FORTY-TWO

He started his journey toward home exactly ten weeks after he sat down to die in our living room.

It was late February by now. The sun had a hint of seductive warmth, fooling no one with its promise but cheering those who held their faces up to it anyway. This time, Jim sat in a wheelchair, carefully propped with fat pillows by Nomita and Elise, the occupational therapist. He did not want this, angrily rejected it. "I don't want to go anywhere," he said. "Please put me back into bed." But Nomita had finally won reluctant concession after nagging him insistently for days. "You need a new perspective," she kept saying, never raising her voice, always reasonable. "You need to see something more than the ceiling."

Jim still resisted, gripping the arm rests. "I'm afraid I might fall out," he said. "I want to go back to bed." But Nomita and Elise quickly improvised a makeshift restraint across his chest, a bed sheet tied in a bulky knot at the back of the wheelchair, under the handles. "Hold yourself up as straight as you can," said Nomita. "That's it. Hold yourself like a king." Then she gave a brief curtsy. "You are a king," she declared.

No, he wasn't, unless she was thinking of Lear. There was nothing majestic about this emaciated man with the long stringy hair and the sunken cheeks and the hands that fidgeted in his lap. This would be the first time he had travelled on anything but a gurney or a bed since admission to hospital. He could not appreciate the significance of the expedition. I could finally recall that first terrible morning without shuddering.

I pushed him cautiously out of the room, just us, turned left and proceeded to the nursing station at the end, trying to get used to the feel of the grips in my hands and the motion of the wheels, the way they wobbled, anxious to keep the chair from rolling forward or sideways when I didn't want it to. We paused while the nurses looked up from their charts to cheer him on, then we made a right turn down a short corridor, past patient rooms filled with strangers who drew no curiosity from him, and we came to rest close to a large window. I set the brakes, remembering instructions from Elise.

At first, all he seemed to see was his reflection in the glass and I realized it was the first time that he had been able to look at himself, that mirrors had been absent from his illness, never requested, never offered. "I'm very skinny," he said.

Then his eyes drifted out from his own image to the backdrop beyond it, a view that swept past the hospital parking lot and the patches of melting snow to a busy thoroughfare. "What's that street?" he asked. I told him it was The Queensway, that it bordered Trillium's north side, so he was looking north now, that it was my route back and forth every day. I did not tell him about my own remembered view of it, four floors down from here, that bleak Christmas Eve when I stood watching the traffic, lighter then than now, and heard a voice tell me "this is not his time" while he was dying upstairs.

I watched him take in the sun and the sky and the snow and the cars and people coming and going below and the buildings across the street bouncing the sun's glare back and the trees stretching into the distance beyond them, and he was a timid tourist blinking at foreign sights. I knew he was overwhelmed and confused by what he was seeing, repelled and tantalized by the enormous, forgotten world outside this cloister. But there was a light in his eyes and I realized it was curiosity, something I had not seen in nearly three months. He placed a hand on the cold glass, held it there for a moment, then removed it. "I think I want to go back to my room now," he said.

He would have to endure five more weeks in hospital — two more weeks on Med 4D and three in a rehabilitation unit. He would have to learn to walk all over again, first supported by someone on each side, then by a large wooden thing like a podium on wheels that he gripped for trips up and down the hospital corridor, triumphantly steering it like a kid practising on his first bike, then pushing a walker, then using two canes, then one cane, and finally, walking with a splint that braced his left lower leg and that sat in our living room for months after he no longer needed it. It made us think of Tiny Tim's abandoned crutches.

He would have to learn to swallow again, enduring noxious stuff whose progress down his throat was visible on a screen monitored by Diana the speech pathologist, a radiologist at her side, their intent to make sure that food would go to his stomach and not to his lungs. It would be a long time before he could enjoy food again, none of his old favourite tastes as satisfying as they had been, and he would carry a fear of choking for months.

He would undergo nearly a year of intensive physiotherapy

and meet a neurologist along the way who would tell him he would never walk normally again and then delight in proving that expert wrong by strapping on his rollerblades for a gleeful tour through the neighbourhood. His bedsores would gradually mend, leaving faded reminders of their presence, and his skin would be patched here and there with odd flashes of white that recalled the tubes and tape attached to him. They would eventually fade too. The tracheotomy incision would take a long time to close, finally leaving a deep round pucker that was reminiscent of a bullet hole. He would hear it called a proud badge of honour by some survivors. He would avoid looking at it every morning when he shaved and then a compassionate surgeon would deftly diminish its presence. But all of the transforming memories of the crisis would linger, emotional scars and insights we would both carry forever, noticeable only to people whose own lives had been brutally altered and then redeemed.

He would eventually keep his promise to Nomita by returning to Trillium Med 4D with a fresh apple pie for her and large tins of home-made cookies for everyone else. Nomita would shake her head and blush. Mabel would pull me to one side. "Good work," she would say and then rejoin her colleagues, all of them looking Jim up and down, assessing him, smiling, obvious and touching in their pleasure at his validating presence.

But that February day with its diffident reach for a world lost for so long was the real beginning of his comeback. I rolled the wheelchair down the hall again, not pausing at the nursing station this time, and Nomita and Elise were waiting for us in his room. I positioned the chair for his expedient transfer back to the bed, and Nomita and Elise moved forward, each ready to take a side of him. But I stopped them. "I'll do this," I said, and I stepped between him and the bed and took him carefully under his arms and lifted him out of the chair so that he was standing, and eased him around so that his back was to the bed, holding him from collapse, and we were joined for that moment in an awkward, shuffling waltz.

Then I paused, just holding him up but closer now, got as close as I could. I was afraid of squeezing him but held him tight anyway, so coupled to him I could feel his chest rise and fall and even feel his heart beating, just like the first night we met, and then his arms slowly lifted and wrapped around me and we stood there, not moving, his head settling on my shoulder, and we were finally us again. "I've waited a long time for this," I whispered. "Me too," he whispered back. Nomita and Elise were silent, each gazing discreetly out the window. After a while, Elise coughed, a mock reproach. "Time's up, you guys. We've got work to do." There were tears in her eyes.

I placed him gently on the edge of the bed, steadied him with one hand while I raised his legs onto the sheet and then lifted him forward and into its centre and organized his pillows under and around him. Nomita and Elise left us alone when they were certain he was safely tucked in again.

We talked about what was away from here, all of it starting to unfold to him again, and I spoke about people and places he still felt unready for, peering at the ceiling to get the names right, of Mary and John and Al and Shirley and Kathy and George and all the nieces and nephews, all of our friends and neighbours, all by name, and about Hope and about my own stuttering loneliness without him and about a garden that would need planting soon and about the characters at the St. Lawrence Market and about Donna from down the street who still felt irrationally guilty over starting all this with a 9-1-1 phone call all those weeks ago, her name still in the dust on the coffee table, my playful scribble when she dropped in for coffee weeks before, more testimony that the house was frozen in time and place, everything suspended until he came home. When I looked down, he was asleep.

I covered him with the thin hospital blanket, checked the tracheotomy dressing at his throat, placed my hand tenderly on his cheek and then sat close to him in the darkening room. His door was open and outside I could hear Mabel crooning to Ted and the distant jangle of the big carts arriving with all the dinner trays and a doctor being paged and Cecilia asking who ordered the double-double coffee and the steady pong of a patient call bell and Catherine laughing at something Heather said and Tina calling for someone's chart, all of the strands weaving into a soundtrack that played softly behind us while he slept and while I waited, both of us peaceful at last in our found communion.

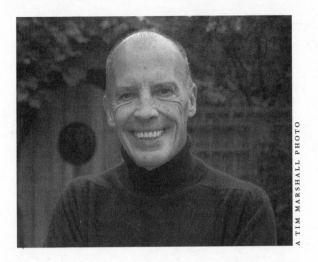

PATRICK CONLON is an award-winning journalist and broadcaster who has written for *Toronto Life*, *Macleans*, the *Globe and Mail* and *The Toronto Star*. From 1990 to 2000, he was host of CBC *Newsworld's* "On the Line," a program that explored controversial issues of the day. He is the author of *Sanctuary: Stories from Casey House Hospice*, a critically acclaimed look at North America's first free-standing hospice for people with AIDS. He is currently leading a groundbreaking initiative to revise Ontario's hospital patient-care model. He lives with Jim, his partner of more than 30 years.

By printing this book on paper made from 100% post-consumer recycled fibre rather than virgin tree fibre, Raincoast Books has made the following ecological savings:

- 26 trees
- 1,019 kilograms of greenhouse gases
- 18 million BTUs of energy
- 2,463 litres of water
- 543 kilograms of solid waste

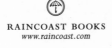

RAINCOAST BOOKS
www.raincoast.com

ANCIENT FOREST
FRIENDLY